Inte   Fasting

The Complete Beginners Guide To Intermittent Fasting For Weight Loss

Cure The Weight Problem And Reverse Chronic Diseases

While Enjoying The Food You Love!

Jason Legg

Table Of Contents

For the horses

Introduction

Psst! Yes you!

Reckon you must be searching for ways to achieve weight loss and somehow you chanced upon this here. First I would like to say a warm welcome to this domain of intermittent fasting and I am absolutely stoked to know that you will be getting loads of value as well as actionable tips with which you can kick start and achieve significant progress on the weight loss journey.

I am by no means the final authority on intermittent fasting, and I would like to say the reason why I felt compelled to share what I know on this subject is because intermittent fasting literally saved my life.

Yes. You can call it a repayment of karmic debt or whatever you would like to term it as because this book as a labor of love is the end result of detailing what I know on intermittent fasting.

To cut the long story short, intermittent fasting was kind of forced upon me when I was diagnosed with all sorts of diseases and syndromes. All at the same time. Metabolic syndrome made its debut in my life, though that wasn't a real surprise considering my bulging waist line. Diabetes paid its call about a month later, and to top everything off, a minor cardiac arrest was the absolute crowning moment in those dark ages. The doctor's advice was to stick to meds and never miss a day. I was of course given the standard prescription for diet, meaning low fat , low calories in order to control weight gain.

It didn't work, and I panicked.

I started to toss aside the usual blind faith that I had in modern medical science and ventured into the world of natural weight loss for solutions to my problems. This and that diet came up, and believe it or not, I once drank olive oil for a straight five days. That was nasty. Eventually and fortuitously, I got hold of the concept of intermittent fasting when one of my neighbors sort of just casually dropped the subject when we were having our little chats. Little did I know it would consume me and I would be blessed once again with great health and a body that did not rely on external medication for proper function.

Intermittent fasting is a subject that has received plenty of widespread attention of late. People who have taken on fasting have managed to achieve some fantastic results in regards to both their health and weight. The phenomena of intermittent fasting is in no way a fad. Fasting has been practiced for centuries now and is considered by many ancient tribes as a means of survival, sacrifice, healing power, and spiritual cleansing. Intermittent fasting is in no way a new eating plan for you to try out for the next few weeks. Intermittent fasting is a way of life.

This book explores the many topics that surround intermittent fasting, such as the various methods of intermittent fasting and the multitude of benefits that have been discovered through numerous studies and research. There are also some useful tips on how to conduct your fast as well as the kind of food you can prepare and eat while taking part in intermittent fasting. The people who practice intermittent fasting today benefit in regards to weight loss and fitness. Studies have also found significant progress in regards to promoting other useful health factors such as inflammation, brain-cell creation, increased energy levels, and mental state. Intermittent fasting also encourages the natural fat-burning state of ketosis, which helps those who fast with shedding belly fat.

Apart from the various health benefits associated with intermittent fasting, you also want to give fasting a try because of a whole host of other reasons. One is the convenience of not having to eat as many meals as you would typically. Intermittent fasting allows you to skip meals, meaning that you will be able to save on the time and cost of preparing meals. Apart from the time and cost savings, you will also be eating much less than you would typically yet not experiencing those darn hunger pangs. This will allow you to automatically control your calorie intake just by following a simple eating timetable promoted by intermittent fasting.

This book goes into specific detail in regards to all of these benefits and how you can implement intermittent fasting to enjoy these benefits. It will help you to drastically improve your life in a healthy way. Intermittent fasting is a superb lifestyle choice and is indeed the way to go.

See you in the fasting nirvana! And oh, please enjoy the weight loss, improved health and better all-around lifestyle while you are in it!

Chapter 1: What is Intermittent Fasting

How Our Modern Diet is a Problem

It is estimated that more than one-third of adults in the United States are obese. This equates to over 78 million people who suffer from obesity. Obesity may be taken lightly by most people, but being obese can increase a person's risk towards certain medical conditions such as diabetes and heart disease. The chances of having a stroke rise in obese individuals. Another alarming statistic regarding obesity is that it is one of the leading causes of preventable death in America.

If you look back at the last few decades, it is possible to find a relationship between the rise in obesity and the way our diets have changed. Not only are we eating mostly processed food, often deep-fried, but we are also consuming larger amounts of food than we used to. The total caloric intake among individuals has gone up by 400 calories per day. The convenience and availability of cheap junk food has made it easily accessible for everyone to consume. However, the disadvantages of this modern diet are overlooked by most people.

The food we eat today is drastically different from the food that was consumed over 40 years ago. Most of the food then was fresh, some of it actually grown at home. Even though there were plenty of diners and fast food outlets back then, people still preferred eating good fresh food at home. In contrast, most of today's food is in some way processed, including the food that you choose to cook at home.

The type of food that we consume today is filled with additives, trans fats, colorings, and other various chemicals and ingredients that were not evident in food just a few decades ago. One of the most significant increases in our modern-day diet is the consumption of sugar. People in America consume 22 teaspoons of sugar on average per day. That makes up for 25 percent of a person's daily caloric intake. If you compare these statistics with past figures, then today's sugar intake has risen 20 percent since the seventies.

People today are obviously not consuming 22 teaspoons of actual sugar. The sugar that we end up consuming is usually found in juices, desserts, and sauces. This processed fructose is also evident in foods that are advertised as being healthy meals. Because of this, many parents will inadvertently give their kids food that's high in sugar.

Another significant contributor towards sugar consumption is soda and fruit juice drinks. Beverages like soda have large amounts of sugar in them and are usually considered as one of the worse sugar sources. Many people who know this tend to skip to a so-called healthier alternative by ordering juice instead of soda. The truth is, juice contains a very similar amount of sugar when compared to soda. And, you guessed it, soda and juice intake has also increased dramatically since the 1970s.

Soda drinks increased in popularity at a rapid rate over the last few decades, peaking around the year 2002. Interest in sodas has dipped ever so slightly since then. However, fruit juice has seen a decent increase in popularity since the late nineties and continues to grow in popularity as compared to the decrease in the popularity of sodas. People seem to be under the general impression that juice is much better for you than soda, but this is false.

If you ever thought of striking out that one thing from the modern diet in order to be healthier, then reducing sugar is the key.

The Food We Consume Today

The type of fats that we consume has also changed over the years. The primary consensus regarding animal fats and other saturated fats is that they can be dangerous for you because they are, most likely, a cause of heart disease. However, vegetable oils, such as corn oil and canola oil, that are processed are so dangerous that recent studies have shown that these daily cooking oils are liable to cause hormonal imbalances and metabolic changes in a person's body.

Repeated use of these oils has also contributed to the current obesity problem. The same can be said for trans fats, which are found in probably every single tasty treat or food in our modern diet. Studies have shown that trans fats, a form of polyunsaturated fats, increase bad LDL cholesterol while not increasing the good HDL cholesterol. Studies show that our use of vegetable oil has significantly increased since the 1960s.

There are also current studies that are focused on the relationship between trans fats and insulin resistance, which drives type 2 diabetes. The sad truth is that, today, many people have replaced heart-healthy butter with margarine that is filled with trans fats.

Some of the types of food that are known to include trans fats are:

- Chocolate
- Margarine
- Ice cream
- Burgers
- Cookies
- Cakes
- Cereals
- Bread
- French fries
- Pizza
- Fried chicken
- Pastries

Even though the consumption of trans fats has been regulated in recent years, we still consume way too much. The consumption of fast foods in the United States has consistently increased at a dramatic rate since the late sixties. A big reason for this is that our go-to food today is processed fast food. We like the convenience of foods that are cooked fast and available to eat on-the-go. No need to prepare a decent breakfast at home when you can fetch a burger at the drive-thru and eat in the car on the way to work. This way, you can get in an extra half hour of work at the office.

This is the perfect solution for productive people. Unfortunately, such food is loaded with trans fats. Even just grabbing snacks from a gas station takes its toll on us. We do this to avoid our hunger during our trip from work to home, instead of just waiting to get home and eat something healthy. These unnecessary processed foods are part of the cause of our terrible modern diet.

The modern diet is the primary reason behind obesity and people becoming sicker than before. More and more people are beginning to adopt the modern diet by abandoning traditional foods in favor of processed food. These processed foods are high in sugar, vegetable oil, and refined flour. On the other hand, eggs are considered to be one of the more nutritious foods out there. Yet our consumption of eggs has also gradually decreased.

Eggs are high in cholesterol, but they do not increase the bad cholesterol in the blood. Nevertheless, people still feel that eggs can cause a negative impact on your cholesterol. Because of this, people began to consume fewer eggs over the course of the years. New studies and diets are more accepting of eggs today and actually promote the consumption of eggs.

The History of Intermittent Fasting

It's clear that intermittent fasting has become something of a popular star today. Apart from the excellent weight-loss results, one of the primary reasons for fasting is the health benefits that one can enjoy. These are some of the elements that have caused intermittent fasting to receive plenty of attention and interest. When people look up intermittent fasting, one of the first things that these people research is the actual origin of intermittent fasting.

Yes, you probably have only recently heard of intermittent fasting, but the truth is, it has been around since ancient times. Back in the time when our ancestors were hunter-gatherers, people used to fast for long periods in between meals. They did this because food back then was not as readily available as it is today.

People used to hunt for food for days until a kill was made. The food that people gathered or claimed during a hunt was then shared over a period of a few days between everyone in the tribe. It was common for people not to find anything for an entire day when out hunting. These people would have to make do with the situation for that day and hope that the next day would be a much more productive day for hunting. If they could not find anything to hunt, then they would search for nuts and fruits that could help sustain them through their tiring hunting sessions.

Our ancestors may have been forced to fast because of their situation in regards to food, but, through fasting, they were able to cope with not having food readily available. Most of the time, these people managed perfectly fine with their fast, as their bodies had adapted to their eating pattern. Their eating pattern assisted in increasing fat oxidation while reducing body weight and accelerating fat loss.

These are some of the benefits that arise from intermittent fasting. Our ancestors didn't fast mostly because of these benefits, but merely as a way of survival. If fasting can be seen as a primary means of survival, then that alone will tell you how beneficial it can be. Another important part about fasting is feasting. What you eat when you do eventually eat is vital in determining the effectiveness of your fast.

Our ancestors made sure not to overdo it when it was time to eat. They ate rationally, to have enough food to go around, as well as to preserve food for more extended periods. They ate just enough food for them to get by. Only two meals a day was more than sufficient for them to remain nourished and healthy. This meant that these people ate enough food to enable their bodies to store the right amount of fat which would be used as a source of energy in the days to come.

This way of eating may seem irregular in today's age, but it was how we used to eat and how our body was designed to consume food. It is considered one of the best ways to help our body maintain itself, which is key to our health and wellbeing. Eating only when needed is the way to go.

Overeating is considered wrong and unnatural. Consuming large amounts of food forces excess fat on the body which leads to an unhealthy lifestyle. Being overweight and unhealthy can also cause a person to develop various diseases. It is known that our ancestors were much stronger than us. Most people back then had stronger bones than even our modern Olympic athletes. Our ancestors achieved their great physical conditions while fasting for long periods of time.

Other ancient civilizations, such as the Ancient Greeks and Egyptians, practiced eating patterns similar to that of intermittent fasting. They endured voluntary starvation with the hopes of allowing their bodies to recover from illness. They also understood the benefits behind fasting and undertook regular fasts so that they could enjoy those benefits.

Ancient Greeks and Egyptians also used intermittent fasting as a means of strengthening the body. These civilizations understood that when a person practices intermittent fasting, he or she becomes more alert and focused. This is due to a fasting person's body being able to release an increased amount of norepinephrine, a chemical that functions in the brain as a hormone and neurotransmitter.

Fasting in the Middle Ages

Intermittent fasting continued to be a part of many civilizations for years. It even managed to spread to other parts of the world. Intermittent fasting became popular during the Middle Ages as people took part in fasts for various reasons, primarily to reap the benefits associated with fasting. The Eastern Orthodox and Roman Catholic churches at the time had a significant influence on the diets of people from the Middle Ages.

The church prohibited meat and other animal products on a few different occasions throughout the year. An example of a specific event when meat was forbidden was during Lent, a period preceding Easter. Lent was also an occasion in which people were required to fast for 40 days. This is symbolic of how Christ fasted for 40 days while in the desert. Apart from Lent, most churches also advised that people should alternate between fasting and feasting.

One of the most popular times to fast was on Fridays. Most of the Christian churches saw fasting as a means of degrading the body while refreshing the soul. Fasting also served as a reminder of the humanity of Christ. Being able to fast meant that you and your body underwent abstinence and self-restraint.

Fasting in Religions

Throughout history, different religions have also practiced intermittent fasting. These religions have been fasting for centuries now. In Judaism, there are several days in the year that are reserved towards fasting. Yom Kippur, the Day of Atonement, is the most well-known full fast as it is a fast that is mentioned in the Torah. The purpose of the fast is to "afflict your soul." This can be seen as a form of repentance. The actual duration of the fast is 25 hours and it begins on the evening before Yom Kippur and after nightfall on the day of Yom Kippur.

Strict rules apply to the fast on Yom Kippur. There is no food at all allowed, not even water. Only the elderly, ill, and pregnant woman are exempt from the fast. Apart from Yom Kippur, there are more holidays and events spread out over the year that are associated with fasting. People are also allowed to engage in a private fast if they so wish, as long as they practice the fast within the set of rules.

In Islam, Muslims also practice fasting during the month of Ramadan. They begin their fast early in the morning, just before sunrise, (or before their morning prayer) and they end their fast in the evening, during sunset. All Muslims must take part in this compulsory fast daily for the 30-day duration of Ramadan until the day of Eid al-Fitr. The entire day of fasting prohibits all kinds of food and drink. Muslims cannot eat anything, nor can they even drink water.

There are various reasons behind fasting in the month of Ramadan. Ramadan is seen as a holy month in which the devil ceases to exist. It is a month in which Muslims are encouraged to practice as many good deeds as possible. One such good deed is the act of performing the Taraweeh prayer in the evening. Fasting is another good deed and is considered a form of abstinence and sacrifice. It is also seen as a means to cleanse the body of any external devices and toxins. Fasting and praying during Ramadan are how Muslims cleanse their bodies and their souls.

The Science of Intermittent Fasting

It makes sense for us to take part in intermittent fasting as our ancestors did for centuries. Some of the reasons why they took part in fasts were for survival and health benefits. Our hunter-gatherer ancestors also took part in intermittent fasting so that they could cope with periods of famine. There is a common argument that it certainly makes evolutionary sense if we, too, undertake similar fasts, as our bodies are designed to cope with such eating habits.

At the moment, there is a large body of research to support the health benefits of intermittent fasting, which is good for both your mind and body. However, the majority of the research has been conducted on animals and not on humans. This is why people are calling for more research and monitoring of individuals that are currently undergoing intermittent fasting. The research that is presently available shows that fasting assists in improving biomarkers of disease, preserves learning and memory functions, and reduces oxidative stress.

These findings are according to Mark Mattson, who is a senior investigator for the National Institute of Aging, a division of the US National Institutes of Health. Mattson conducted studies centered around the health benefits of intermittent fasting on the cardiovascular system and brain within rodents. In his studies, Mattson developed several theories about why fasting provides physiological benefits.

One interesting theory is that, during the fasting period, our cells are under mild stress. Because of this, our cells then respond by adapting to that stress. Our cells accomplish this by enhancing their ability to cope with stress and possibly enhancing themselves in order to resist disease more effectively. The stress that our cells may undergo during fasting does sound negative, but this type of stress can be comparable to the stress that our body undergoes during intense workout sessions in the gym or other vigorous exercise.

These sorts of high-intensity workouts place high levels of stress on your muscles and cardiovascular system. If you spend the right amount of time allowing your body to recover afterward, then your body will become stronger over time. Mattson says that there is a similarity between how our cells respond to the stress of exercise and how our cells respond to intermittent fasting.

Mattson has contributed to a specific study in which overweight adults with moderate asthma consumed only 20 percent of their daily caloric intake on alternate days. This meant that the subjects would perform a fast on one day, then eat normally the next day, then fast again the day after, and so on. The findings were that those who adhered to the diet managed to lose nine percent of their initial body weight over the course of eight weeks. Mattson also found a decrease in stress and inflammation, with an improvement of asthma-related symptoms and overall health.

In other studies, Mattson also explored the effects of intermittent fasting and energy restriction on weight loss and other biomarkers among young overweight woman. These biomarkers included conditions such as diabetes, breast cancer, and cardiovascular disease. The findings were that intermittent restriction was as effective as a continuous dietary restriction to improve weight loss. The results were just as positive towards insulin sensitivity and other health biomarkers.

Ketosis

Mattson also undertook studies of how fasting is related to neurons. He found that if you don't eat for 10 to 16 hours, then your body will begin to use its fat stores for energy. When this happens, then the fatty acids known as ketones get released into the bloodstream. This process has been shown to protect memory and functionality as well as to slow down disease processes in the brain.

Continuously fasting while on a low-carb diet allows your body to enter the state of ketosis. Ketosis occurs when your body switches over from its primary energy source, glucose, to another source of energy, known as ketones. As mentioned earlier, ketones are produced from the fat stores in our body. When our body runs out of glucose (or blood sugar), which mostly comes from the carbohydrates that we eat, then it will rely on ketones for energy.

The consensus is that when a person's body is in ketosis, then he or she will have to burn fat faster to consistently generate the ketones required for energy. If you wish to achieve a state of ketosis, then you will have to force your body not to produce any more glucose. A way of doing this is just to cut out carbs. Low-carb diets, such as the ketogenic diet, promote the state of ketosis by cutting daily carb intake to only five percent, overall, and increasing fat intake to 75 percent.

The keto diet makes it possible to have few to no carbs daily with increased consumption of fats. This means that your body will not have any more carbs to turn into glucose for energy. Instead, your body will rely on the fats you consume. This way, your body will remain in the fat-burning state of ketosis. Another way of achieving ketosis is through intermittent fasting.

Fasting for long periods of time means that your body will run out of its default source of energy, which is glucose. This means that while you are fasting, it will be possible for your body to transition to burning excess fat for fuel. Many people who practice the ketogenic diet on a daily basis also undergo intermittent fasting. The reason for this is that both promote the fat-burning state of ketosis very well.

It is important to remember that your body does not simply switch over into ketosis after just a single day of fasting. The process is long and can take up to seven days. In that time you will have had to watch the amount of carbs you ate which turn into glucose, while consuming the correct amount of fats that will be converted to ketones, to sustain yourself. Taking in large amounts of protein, instead of fats, will not work as our bodies will also convert excess protein into glucose.

Why You Want to Fast

The most common reason why a person wants to fast is to lose weight. If you do have issues with weight or you want to shape up a bit to fit into that gorgeous dress, then successfully implementing intermittent fasting into your life can be a way to achieve all of this. However, weight loss isn't the only reason you should be fasting. There are many other health reasons why you should fast. These are possibly some of the benefits that our ancestors enjoyed when they went on their periodic fasts.

Another excellent reason for why you should fast is that intermittent fasting is a natural calorie restriction method. You will notice that your caloric intake will automatically go down when you begin fasting, as long as you don't overdo your meals during your eating window. Let's take a more in-depth look at the benefits behind intermittent fasting.

The Benefits of Fasting

In recent times, people have begun to realize that there are plenty of benefits that one can enjoy while taking part in intermittent fasting. Some of the benefits include general food and caloric restrictions that can help promote weight loss as well as creating opportunities to skip meals. Not having to cook individual meals on a daily basis can directly equate to less effort in preparing meals as well as time and money savings.

If you plan to skip breakfast entirely on a daily basis, then you can save up on the expenses related to your first meal of the morning. It also means that you no longer need to wake up earlier to prepare your breakfast in the mornings before you rush off to work. You can now allocate your time in the morning for other activities. Apart from time and money savings, there are a few other benefits that you can enjoy while taking up intermittent fasting.

Weight Loss

Most people who take up intermittent fasting today are doing so to lose weight. If done correctly, intermittent fasting will allow you to eat fewer meals per day. This will drop your overall caloric intake. Apart from this, intermittent fasting enhances hormone function and facilitates weight loss. This is achieved through higher growth-hormone levels, lower insulin levels, and increased amounts of norepinephrine. These are the defining factors that assist the body in breaking down body fat to use it for energy.

Because of this, short-term fasting will increase your metabolic rate by up to 14 percent. That means that you will be able to burn even more calories on a daily basis. So if you are someone that pays careful attention to calories, then intermittent fasting has you covered on both sides. This is because intermittent fasting will force you to consume fewer calories while increasing your metabolic rate, helping you to burn those calories faster.

Research has shown that intermittent fasting over a period of three to 24 weeks causes people to lose between three to eight percent of their weight. People also managed to lose between four to seven percent of their waist circumference, meaning that they managed to lose plenty of belly fat. This is a massive benefit as belly fat is considered to be harmful fat in the abdominal cavity that can cause diseases. Studies have also shown that intermittent fasting will not cause you to lose as much muscle mass as a continuous caloric restriction.

Fitness

There are plenty of people who avoid intermittent fasting as they feel it will cause their fitness levels to deteriorate. This isn't necessarily the case for those people who do take part in intermittent fasting, as studies have shown that fasting does not negatively impact those who perform regular physical activities, especially if you cut down on your carbs as you fast and are in a ketosis state. Studies have shown that physical training while fasting can lead to higher metabolic adaptations.

Higher metabolic adaptations mean that your performance can increase in the long run. Taking part in physical training while fasting can also improve your body's response to post-workout meals. Consuming your pre-workout meal during your feasting periods will cause your body to absorb the nutrients even faster. This can lead to improved results. If you consume the proper nutrients, train the right way, and stick to regular fasts, then it is still possible to expect good muscle gains.

Reduces Inflammation

Excessive inflammation in our bodies can lead to many other chronic diseases such as dementia, Alzheimer's disease, diabetes, and more. Inflammation takes place in our bodies when white blood cells, and all of the other substances that they produce, begin to protect us from harmful bacteria and viruses. This sort of inflammation is necessary to dismiss any harmful bacteria. However, diseases, such as arthritis, trigger the very same inflammatory response even when there is no threat. These autoimmune diseases force the body's immune system to cause damage to its tissues as if it were trying to protect the body from a virus.

Intermittent fasting promotes autophagy, a process in which the body destroys its old or damaged cells. Killing off old cells may sound like a terrible notion. However, it can be seen as a way of removing old and unwanted dirt from your body. It's a simple method for the body to clean and repair itself. Old and damaged cells can create inflammation. Because intermittent fasting stimulates autophagy, then it is possible to reduce inflammation in your body while fasting.

When a person is fasting, their body ends up using all of its blood sugar stores because there is not food entering the body. Their body will then have to turn to fat for fuel. When this happens, the fat stores in the body get broken down further into ketones. Some ketones, such as hydroxybutyrate, block part of the immune system that is responsible for the regulation of inflammatory disorders such as arthritis and Alzheimer's.

When a person's body becomes insulin resistant, insulin and glucose build up in the blood, which then goes on to create inflammation. Fasting is known to assist in resolving insulin resistance. When a person is taking part in intermittent fasting, they are allowing their body to have a break from digesting foods. Because there is no food being consumed, the body will end up using all of its sugar stores, causing insulin levels to drop. Such a process can allow the body to re-sensitize itself again to insulin.

Burns Fat for Fuel

Studies have shown that fat is a cleaner and better source of energy than carbohydrates. Fat is known to produce more energy per gram than carbs do. This is probably why people on low-carb diets can control their hunger. Fats are also known to produce less free radicals during the energy-burning process. These free radicals are one of the causes of inflammation.

Free radicals are a form of waste that gets produced when your mitochondria (the body's battery cells) use carbs or fats to burn energy. Free radicals are also known to cause oxidative stress in the body. They are thought to be a cause of many other chronic diseases such as neurodegenerative diseases. Intermittent fasting also allows your brain to use ketones which are derived from fat, rather than sugar. Ketones are known to be a cleaner and more efficient fuel for your brain.

Brain-Cell Creation

Dr. Mark Mattson has found in his studies that fasting can increase the rates of neurogenesis in the brain. Neurogenesis is the development and growth of new brain cells and nerve tissues. This means that fasting can indeed assist you in creating more brain cells which will, therefore, improve your brain power. People who have higher rates of neurogenesis are known to have increased brain performance, focus, mood, and memory. Some studies show that intermittent fasting stimulated the production of new brain cells.

Increased Energy Levels

Fasting boosts neurogenesis as well as mitochondrial biogenesis. As mentioned earlier, neurogenesis is associated with the growth and development of new brain cells and nerve tissues. Mitochondrial biogenesis has to do with the creation of new mitochondria, which are known as the body's batteries for its cells. Each cell in your body has hundreds of mitochondria that power the cells to do their job.

Mitochondria in the brain are known to assist your brain in having more brain power. Fasting promotes brain power, which means that people who fast won't feel lazy and tired in the long run. Instead, they will be energetic and focused.

Mental State

Our brains are massive consumers of energy. Fats that are processed into ketones are considered to be the best energy-efficient fuel to run your brain and your body effectively. This means that your brain can continuously run on fuel that is derived from the fat that is stored in your body. It is even possible to use the fat that you consume as fuel. Using a preferred and effective energy source to power your brain can leave you feeling more focused and energetic.

When some people are under stress, they tend to turn to carbs as a way of seeking some form of release. Eating sweet or starchy food that contains carbs will allow the brain to make new serotonin. Serotonin makes us feel calmer, which in turn makes us feel as if we can cope. When fasting, your body will rely mostly on your fat stores for energy, meaning that you won't feel the need to snack on carbs to cope with mental fatigue or stress.

Muscle During Intermittent Fasting

There have been recent studies focused on the effects of

intermittent fasting on males. One particular study was centered around the impact that 16-hour intermittent fasting had on men who were lifting weights in the gym. The study found that their muscle mass remained very much the same while their fat mass decreased significantly. The best results were achieved within the group that fasted for 16 hours as opposed to the group that fasted for just 12 hours.

People who are physically active and spend plenty of time in the gym are reluctant to take on intermittent fasting, as they feel that going on for long periods of time without food will, in fact, cause them to lose muscle mass. This is apparently not true, as per various recent studies. One particular study surprisingly showed that, when combining resistance training with 20 hours of fasting, the results were an actual increase in muscle mass, strength, and even endurance.

The subjects in that study only consumed about 650 calories per day. Some studies have also shown that untrained and overweight individuals benefit from intermittent fasting when comparing their muscle and weight-loss statistics to other individuals who just cut down their caloric intake. Undergoing extended periods of fasting has been proven to be more reliable than eating anytime while restricting calories.

The Benefits of Ketosis

Diets such as the keto diet were developed in the past as a way to treat people with neurological diseases such as epilepsy. Such a diet was meant for people who had difficulties controlling their epilepsy. The purpose of this was to promote the state of ketosis within those people who had epilepsy. Studies have shown that ketones aid in reducing the frequency of a person's epileptic seizures.

Similar studies have also shown that more than half of the people who are suffering from epilepsy managed to lessen the frequency of seizures by around half while on a diet that promotes ketosis. These exceptional results continued even after the subjects were taken off their diet.

There have been more studies that highlight the benefits associated with ketosis. Ketosis works well with controlling symptoms related to heart disease. Some of these symptoms are body fat, cholesterol levels, and blood sugar. At the present moment, people who are currently suffering from cancer and slow tumor growth are being advised to consider the ketogenic diet. The diet itself is not a means of curing the disease, but it serves as a means of making use of the advantages that are associated with ketosis.

Those who have studied ketosis have so far given a positive response to the advantages that are associated with it. Not only has there been a positive response concerning neurological studies, but there have been studies on the effects of ketosis on other health conditions, most of which have seen some positive results as well. Various researchers and medical practitioners are currently researching ketosis and its effects on the following medical conditions:

- Heart disease

- Epilepsy

- Acne

- Alzheimer's disease

- Parkinson's disease

- Polycystic ovary syndrome

- Brain injuries

This type of research has raised questions regarding intermittent fasting and ketosis and their application throughout history and various cultures. Many cultures and civilizations used to undergo intermittent fasts when they were ill or injured. People used fasting as a means of treating illness. The science and research was not as advanced as now, but the people back then already knew of the significant benefits of intermittent fasting and ketosis.

Chapter 2: Meet The Family

There are a few different approaches that one can take when practicing intermittent fasting. Taking on intermittent fasting does not mean that you are fully restricted to just a single method of fasting. In fact, you can select a method that best suits you and your lifestyle. All of the different intermittent-fasting methods are regarded as being useful by those people who have implemented them into their lives.

It is advised that you test out as many different methods as you can when you begin your intermittent-fasting journey. Some methods may not seem enticing to you on paper, but when put into practice, they may be the most suitable method. Not everyone experiences intermittent fasting the same way. This is due to certain lifestyle choices. Physically active people may not adapt to a specific fasting method in the exact same way that other non-active people do.

When it comes down to food, anything goes during your eating window. Most methods of intermittent fasting are more focused on the timing of your meals instead of the actual meals themselves. However, it is advisable to eat normally during your eating window. If you overdo it during these times, then you will have simply made up for the time that you did not eat. This will render the fast useless, especially if you really went all out and consumed more food than you would typically have consumed without fasting.

Intermittent fasting is not considered to be a dry fast. This means that you are allowed to drink water or coffee while you are fasting. During a dry fast, you are strictly prohibited from eating or drinking anything, including water. This isn't the case with intermittent fasting. There are people that actually drink low-calorie supplements while they are fasting.

If you do plan to take your diet and intermittent fasting seriously, then it is also advisable to stick to a low-carb diet. This way, you will not allow carbs to re-enter your body during times when you are feasting. That way your body will continue to remain in a state of ketosis, even while you are eating. Diets such as the ketogenic diet promote ketosis. This is because these diets are high fat, low carb-diets that focus on maintaining a fat-burning state within your body.

The 16/8 Method

This method will require you to fast every day, for around 16 hours. If you manage to accomplish this, then you will have restricted yourself to eating for only eight hours in the day. You will still be able to fit in about two to three meals within this eight-hour window. The easiest way to accomplish this method is to skip breakfast while refraining from eating anything after dinner.

No breakfast and no food after dinner roughly translates to having your first meal of the day at noon, with your last meal of the day at 8 p.m., just after supper. If you prefer to have your supper earlier, at around 6 p.m., then you can treat that supper as your last meal of the day. You can then have an early night and begin your day with your first meal at 10 a.m. It's best to adjust your eating times according to your lifestyle.

It's best to schedule your fasting times around the time you sleep. You naturally do not consume food while you are asleep.

So the time that you sleep can be considered as part of your fasting time. If your sleep goal is eight hours per day, then perhaps schedule your fast to begin four hours before you sleep and to end four hours after you have woken up.

The 16/8 Method was initially made famous by fitness expert Martin Berkhan. The term that is currently associated with this fasting method is the Leangains protocol. This is the name that people from the world of fitness and nutrition use when discussing the 16/8 method of intermittent fasting. An example of an eating plan for this fast is as follows:

- 12 p.m. – Breakfast

- 4 p.m. – Second Meal

- 8 p.m. – Last Meal

Those who workout professionally or casually with weights can adjust meals according to their preference, as long as they are eating only within the available window. If you workout at around noon, then you can just have a pre-workout meal before you workout. Your biggest meal of the day can be after your workout, around 1 p.m.

Try not to feel discouraged about losing muscle mass when you do go for more extended periods without food. As mentioned before, studies have shown that intermittent fasting does not contribute to the loss of muscle mass. If you are someone who goes to bed early, then adjust the times of your eating window from 10 a.m. to 6 p.m. Once you have become comfortable with this eating plan, you can then adjust it further to shorten your eating window from eight hours to, say, seven hours.

The opposite applies in the case when you feel that eight hours may seem too much for you to adapt to right away. You can bump your eating window to nine hours. The purpose of doing this shouldn't be to consume more food, but rather because you wish to adapt your new intermittent- fasting method to your lifestyle gradually. An example would be those who are only allowed to eat at 10 a.m. at their workplace, and just get to have supper at 7 p.m.

If your lifestyle only permits you to eat at the above-mentioned times, leaving your eating window at nine hours, you can adjust to having your first meal at 1 p.m., but this may leave you feeling way too hungry in the morning. This can be discouraging for you, especially if you are busy at work with an empty stomach. It is okay to start off the 16/8 method of intermittent fasting with a nine-hour eating window. As the weeks go by, you may begin to enjoy the fast to a point where you will start trying to adjust your lifestyle and eating pattern to an eating window that's around eight hours or less.

Some people have their first meal early in the morning, at 6 a.m., which is around the time they wake up. These people stop all forms of eating at around 2 p.m. This fits in well with the 16/8 method of intermittent fasting as they are fasting for the full 16 hours, from 2 p.m. in the afternoon till 6 a.m. the next day. There is absolutely nothing wrong with this method of fasting. However, it can be challenging to keep up with social commitments that require you to have dinner with friends or family. Cutting off eating at 2 p.m. means no afternoon snacks or dinner.

Most people still feel more comfortable with merely avoiding to eat in the mornings. Not only is it more convenient, but it allows you the opportunity to have a good meal in the evening with your family. Also, eating in the afternoon and evening is a great way to relax from a hard day of work. Using up your eight-hour eating window in the morning means that you will not be able to eat in the evening and may possibly miss out on lunch as well. Not being able to enjoy supper and lunch with friends and family may discourage you from fasting.

The recommended fasting window for women is around 14 to 15 hours. This is about the estimated time that woman should fast to achieve the best results. When it comes to achieving the best results from the 16/8 fast, everyone should try and stick to a healthy diet and not overdo it when eating during the eight-hour eating window. Consuming large amounts of carbs or junk food during your eating window can make it difficult for you to fast the next day. Large amounts of carbs can leave you feeling hungry during periods when you are not eating.

It's best to practice a low-carb diet that can assist you in remaining full and satisfied during and after your eating window. Taking in too many carbs can also deprive your body of staying in a fat- burning ketosis state. The 16/8 method of fasting is also one of the most popular methods of intermittent fasts because it is the most natural kind of fasting method out there. Because the 16/8 intermittent-fasting method feels so natural, it has become one of the most straightforward and natural methods to adopt as it requires you to practice the fast daily, making it easier to adopt the new eating habit. It is perfect for beginners who wish to start their journey into intermittent fasting.

The 5:2 Diet

The 5:2 intermittent fast requires you to eat normally for five days of the week and to regulate your caloric intake for two days. The estimated caloric intake for the two days should be around 500 to 600 calories per day. Men on this fast can consume about 600 calories on each of the fasting days and women should stick to 500 calories. Probably the best way to achieve this is to have two light meals of around 250 to 300 calories on the days you choose to fast.

The 5:2 diet has become one of the more popular methods of intermittent fasting of late. This is because the fast allows you some flexibility. You will only be required to dedicate two days a week towards fasting. This makes it easier for people to schedule their lives accordingly. An example would be not to commit to lunch meetings with friends on the days that you are fasting. It is also just two days in the week in which you will have to say no to a person who is offering you something to eat.

Saying no to someone who is offering you food seems like an incredibly trivial problem. However, it can become a nuisance after a while as you have to always explain yourself to people by telling them why you are fasting. There's no issue when it comes to talking about intermittent fasting. But it can be distracting when someone new is trying to understand your eating habits while you are at work. If you chose to fast daily with the 16/8 method, chances are someone at work is going to ask "why you are not eating" in the mornings.

Monday and Thursday are the most common days to take part in the 5:2 intermittent-fasting method. There is no restriction as to when you should fast. However, these days are generally the ideal days for most people to fast. The most important rule regarding the days that you fast is that there must be at least one day in between the two fasting days. So you can select Monday and Wednesday as your two days to fast as long as you keep your caloric restrictions to a minimum on those two days.

As with most fasts, for the fasts to be effective, it is best to maintain moderate consumption of food during the periods when you are not fasting. If your first meal after your fast is a large, carb-heavy and unhealthy meal, then you will be rendering the fast t useless. Don't overcompensate during times when you do eat. Try to eat as you would normally eat when practicing a healthy and balanced diet.

There haven't been too many studies focused on the benefits of the 5:2 method. Yet, people, in general, feel that this method is a much better and natural choice over other kinds of calorie- restriction diets. One of the big reasons for this is that the 5:2 method is easier to implement in any individual's lifestyle. Intermittent fasting, in general, has its benefits even when practiced twice a week.

A 24-Hour Fast – Eat-Stop-Eat

The Eat-Stop-Eat method of intermittent fasting is just a single 24-hour fast that takes place at least once a week, as long as it is in between regular eating days. Going without food for an entire day is in no way an easy feat, but it is achievable. Some people actually practice this fast twice a week. To these people, it is almost like the 5:2 method of intermittent fasting, except for the fact that, instead of restricting calories, they don't eat anything at all.

The Eat-Stop-Eat method of intermittent fasting was made famous by fitness expert Brad Pilon. Taking part in a 24-hour fast usually means fasting from dinner on one day right up to dinner the next day. If you eat your dinner at 7 p.m., then that will be the time you begin your fast. As with the other fasts, no eating is allowed, except for water and coffee, right up until dinner the next evening. So you begin fasting after dinner at 7 p.m. and end your fast with dinner the next day, at 7 p.m.

You can adjust the times according to your lifestyle or schedule. Examples would be to fast from breakfast to breakfast or from lunch to lunch. However, it is important to adhere to a full 24- hour day of fasting. It is absolutely crucial that you make sure you have a normal, healthy supper the evening that you break your fast. It is easy to get tempted into preparing large meals while you are fasting. Your hunger can easily trick you into craving more food than you actually require.

It is important not to overcompensate when eating after you have performed your 24-hour fast. If you do eat much more than you usually would, then the fast will not have been a successful one. Try to stick to regular healthy eating habits and do your best to regulate your appetite. The Eat-Stop-Eat method of intermittent fasting is considered to be a popular method of fasting for many people. However, this method has its flaws.

With the Eat-Stop-Eat method, you are required to go without food for an entire day, which can prove to be difficult for most people. And because this fast only needs to be done once a week, it will take much longer for someone to adapt to this method. If you do wish to start off with this method, due to convenience, and you are having difficulties enduring a full-day fast, then you can begin with 16-hour fasts. Fast from dinner up until lunch the next day, then gradually increase your fasting window until you are ready to go a full day.

Alternate-Day Fasting

The alternate-day fasting method requires you to fast every other day. One day to eat, one day to fast, then the next day is to eat, and so on. The alternate-day fasting method is seen as a more advanced method of intermittent fasting. That is why it certainly isn't recommended for beginners. It's best for beginners to start off their intermittent fasting journey by merely fasting for small periods of time before they feel they are ready to take on more advanced methods such as this one.

During alternate-day fasting, you must fast an entire 24-hour day on the day of your fast. No food permitted, except for water and coffee. The alternate-day method is similar to the Eat-Stop-Eat method, in which you practice a full 24-hour fast. The big difference is that instead of just undergoing a single day of fasting per week, you have three to four full fasting days a week. This method may seem extreme, but it is achievable. There are variations of this method that allow you to consume about 500 calories during the days when you fast.

As with all of the other methods of intermittent fasting, it is imperative that you eat a normal, healthy diet on the days that you are not fasting. Overcompensating during these days will cause your body to make up for the days that it did not consume any food. This will be a massive waste on your part and will not make your fast effective enough to help you lose weight quickly.

The Warrior Diet

The Warrior Diet requires you to fast each and every day. However, you are allowed one large meal at the end of the day. This means no food the entire day, just water and coffee as usual, but a big meal at the end of the day to break your fast. There are other versions of the Warrior Diet that allow room for small portions of raw fruit and vegetables during the day while you are fasting. During the evening, you are allowed a single large meal within a four-hour eating window.

The Warrior Diet was one of the first methods of intermittent fasting to be popularized in recent times. Ori Hofmekler famously used this method of intermittent fasting. The type of food that is recommended for this diet is closely associated with the Paleo Diet. The food consumed is mostly unprocessed, with some fruits allowed.

Spontaneous Meal-Skipping

Spontaneous meal-skipping allows you the opportunity to take part in unplanned or unscheduled fasting periods in your life. The purpose of this is to unofficially fast by skipping meals in the hopes of enjoying some of the benefits associated with intermittent fasting. It is as simple as skipping meals from time to time. Some examples would be to skip breakfast and hold out until lunch, or to have a decent-sized breakfast and then fast until dinner.

If you do decide to skip out on lunch, only to eat dinner later on, then it is important to remember, once again, not to overdo it at dinnertime. Eating more than usual, due to your hunger, will add unnecessary calories to your daily intake. This is not what you want, especially if you have held out on calories during lunchtime.

P.S

If you have found any one thing of value or something which you have benefited from in this book so far, could I please seek your help here to leave a review over in Amazon

It would be super helpful to let more folk know about what was the one thing that you learnt or benefited from

Thank You Very Much !

How to Start Fasting

Apart from the various methods of intermittent fasting available, there are also different types of fasts available. The kind of fast you choose should be based on whatever it is you are trying to achieve as well as how you wish to approach your fast. Here are a few common types of fasts that are practiced today.

Water Fasting

This fast allows you only to consume water while you are fasting. If you take on the 5:2 method of fasting, then you can restrict yourself to just drinking water on the two days of the week when you fast. Some people include coffee as well, which is acceptable. Being able to drink water during the day may not seem like fasting to some people, but having water can help with bad breath and can keep you hydrated.

Juice Fasting

This fast allows you to consume either vegetable or fruit juice. Also known as juice cleansing, it's a diet that requires you to abstain from solid food consumption. Most people use juice fasting as a means of detoxification, which can be seen as an alternative medicine treatment. This method has seen plenty of criticism, as people usually go for days, and sometimes weeks, without food. Some people perform a juice fast as a way to detox for seven days.

This isn't the way to go as it can be potentially dangerous to your health by causing muscle loss, with the possibility of regaining even more fat once the detox has ended. There is also a significant amount of sugar in fruit juices. If you blend fruits yourself, there still will be plenty of sugar in the juice that you blend. If you plan to fast to lose weight, it's best to keep away from juices and stick to a healthy low-carb diet.

Partial Fasting

Partial fasting offers some benefits similar to intermittent fasting. However, the effects of the fast and detox will be slower than normal intermittent fasting. Partial fasting is also known as selective fasting, a cleansing diet, and a modified diet, to name a few. This type of fast is similar to spontaneous fasting in which people set fasting goals that they need to stick to.

Calorie Restriction

Calorie restriction is a common way for people to regulate their eating habits to lose weight. Intermittent fasting can be seen as a form of calorie restriction as your eating window is now much smaller than it used to be, restricting the amount of food that you will consume.

To get started with fasting, it's best that you experiment with the various methods and types of fasting available. The easiest method is the spontaneous meal-skipping method, and one of the most difficult methods is the alternate-day fast. Spontaneous meal-skipping can be a great way for you to get used to skipping meals such as lunch or supper. This way, you will gradually begin to get a sense of what it feels like to fast.

In some cases, while practicing spontaneous meal-skipping correctly and frequently, you may actually begin to reap some of the benefits of intermittent fasting, such as adequate calorie restriction, which in turn assists you in losing weight. Once you begin to start gaining confidence in not eating for long durations of time, you can then take on intermittent fasting for longer durations on a daily basis.

Abstaining from food can be difficult to achieve. The reason for this is that we are so accustomed to eating whenever we want. A person who fasts has a different mindset altogether. There is no temptation for food, just a focus on getting through the fast. The added benefits of intermittent fasting should replace the temptation for food. Instead of thinking about your next meal, think about how your fast is going to benefit you by helping you to lose weight.

Once you are used to fasting and have developed a good fasting mindset, then you can start taking on more advanced intermittent-fasting methods such as the 16/8 method or the 5:2 method. The 16/8 method is easy to implement into anyone's lifestyle. This method requires you to skip one meal only (such as breakfast). In doing so, you will drop your eating window to just eight hours.

The truth behind a smaller eating window is that you have to cut out some food from your daily intake, the most apparent food being junk food. If you are a person who snacks throughout the night, you will automatically have to ditch your midnight snacks to fast effectively. If you plan on keeping your junk food snacks, then they will have to replace real food. The last thing that you want is to be eating only junk food in place of any real food.

If a straight 16-hour daily fast is difficult at first for you, then perhaps try to fast for 12 to 13 hours per day. You could begin your fast at 6 p.m. and end your fast at 6 a.m. You will be asleep for most of the time, which will make your fast much easier to handle. If you are someone that likes to snack after six, you will have to try and cut out the snacks altogether or reserve a portion of your snacks for during the day.

Once you feel you have found a good routine, especially in regards to eating at night, you can then extend your fast a little further by only eating in the morning at 7 a.m., instead of 6 a.m. This will give you an extra hour of fasting. You can then push yourself further, right up to 10 a.m., to enjoy a full 16-hour fast. The 16/8 intermittent fast method is perfect for those who are trying to establish a good routine because this method requires you to fast daily. Implementing a daily fast will help you to develop a good habit towards fasting quickly.

The same cannot be entirely said about the 5:2 fast. It may be a bit more difficult to form a routine around this fast as you are only required to fast twice a week. On the other five days, your daily lifestyle and routine are the same. So, on these days, there's no proper detachment from your old lifestyle, with no sign of your new fasting lifestyle that is only reserved for other days. It's not that the 5:2 method is unachievable; it will just take a bit longer for most people. It's best to work your way to this more advanced method by trying out the 16/8 method, as mentioned above.

The alternate-day fast is meant for the seasoned pros who have gotten the act of intermittent fasting down to a science (just a figure of speech here). This method requires a full-day fast every other day. Yes, it is recommended for pros only, but you can still work your way up to this point and take on this fasting method once you are ready. Many average people take part in consecutive fasts because of their religion or culture. It is possible that you can achieve the alternate-day fasting method.

As with the rest of the methods, take your time and gradually work your way into the alternate- day fasting method. Fast for half days on your fast days, then implement heavy calorie restrictions, of around 500 calories, once you are ready. It is critical always to remember to eat normally and conservatively when you are not fasting and not to overdo it in a way that will overcompensate for the time you spent not eating.

It is also important to remember that you should see a doctor first before getting into fasting if you suffer from any medical condition. If you are a woman and you find yourself undergoing uncomfortable symptoms as a result of fasting, then it is best that you stop fasting and consult your GP. Women are advised to fast for shorter durations at first, for their bodies to appropriately adapt to fasting.

Fasting for General Health

Intermittent fasting, or any form of fasting, has been shown to have a host of different health benefits ranging from better brain function to general weight loss. Studies have found that fasting may assist in improving blood sugar control. This is something that can prove to be useful for those people who are at risk for diabetes. One study, in particular, required ten people with type 2 diabetes to take on short-term intermittent fasting. The fasting managed to decrease the participant's blood sugar levels.

Another study that was based on alternate-day fasting found that this method of fasting was just as effective at limiting calorie intake as it was at reducing insulin resistance. If you manage to decrease the insulin resistance in your body, then you will increase your body's sensitivity to insulin. This will allow your body to transport glucose from your bloodstream to your cells more efficiently.

Fasting has the potential for lowering blood sugar in most people. This can be seen as a great way to keep blood sugar steady, while preventing any spikes in blood sugar levels. It is important to remember that blood sugar level results can differ among individuals, especially between men and women. The results that one person may experience can be entirely different from a woman who might experience adverse effects on her blood sugar levels while fasting.

Intermittent fasting has the potential to enhance heart health. Fasting can have positive effects on a person's blood pressure, cholesterol levels, and triglycerides. One of the easiest and most recommended ways to reduce your risk of heart disease is to change up your current diet and lifestyle for a healthier diet. Research has shown that fasting on a regular basis can be beneficial, especially when it comes to heart health.

Studies have found that fasting can naturally increase human growth hormone (HGH) levels. HGH is a protein type that is related to many aspects regarding your health. Some of the aspects include metabolism, weight loss, growth, and muscle strength. One study, in particular, tested 11 healthy adults who had just fasted for 24 hours. The results showed that these adults were left with significantly increased levels of HGH.

Research (mostly limited to animals) shows that intermittent fasting can assist by boosting brain function (or brain health) and can even go as far as preventing neurodegenerative disorders. One study, in particular, showed that mice who practiced intermittent fasting for 11 months had improved brain structure and brain function. Another study based on animals showed that intermittent fasting can protect brain health. The same study also showed that fasting assists in increasing the generation of nerve cells which are used to help enhance cognitive function.

Others studies that were conducted on animals suggest that intermittent fasting can protect and even improve health conditions such as Alzheimer's disease or Parkinson's. Intermittent fasting is well known for being able to relieve inflammation. Because of this, fasting may also aid in preventing neurodegenerative disorders. Most of the studies that are undertaken towards animals have brought positive results in regards to intermittent fasting. However, there is still a need for studies to accurately analyze the effects that fasting can have on a human's brain.

More animal-based studies have yielded positive results in regards to extended lifespan as a result of fasting. A study has shown that rats that fasted every other day delayed their rate of aging. These rats managed to live 83 percent longer than other rats that did not fast. There have been other similar reports from animal studies that found that fasting can be effective in increasing longevity, as well as survival rates.

Speed Up Metabolism

A recent study found that people who successfully practice the 5:2 method of intermittent fasting manage to lower their risk of heart disease as well as attain a faster metabolism when compared to other groups that used older calorie-counting methods of restricting food consumption. These people didn't change their diets substantially by cutting down on carbs. They simply made sure that they performed their two fasts weekly.

On a weekly basis, after fasting for two days, you will have consumed fewer calories in that week as compared to not having fasted at all. However, this is only accomplished if you perform the fasts correctly and don't overeat on the non-fast days. It is advisable to have around 500 calories on the days that you fast. This should be sufficient to keep you going for the rest of the day.

Fasting for Weight Loss

Intermittent fasting can be seen as an effective way to reduce calories, which in turn can assist you in losing weight. Fasting on a regular basis will ensure that you consume fewer calories overall. If you successfully skip meals while maintaining normal eating patterns while you are not fasting, then your calorie intake should be well regulated. If you overcompensate by overeating during times when you are not fasting, then you may still be consuming the same amount of calories that you would have before fasting.

A 2014 study found that intermittent fasting can, in fact, lead to significant weight loss. The study states that intermittent fasting managed to help people reduce body weight by three to eight percent over a period of three to 24 weeks. A more in-depth look into the weight-loss figures showed that people who performed regular intermittent fasting lost about 0.25 kg/0.55 pounds per week. People who took part in alternate-day fasting actually lost 0.75 kg/1.65 pounds per week. People also managed to lose belly fat. The loss totaled between four to seven percent of a person's waist circumference.

Intermittent fasting methods are natural ways of sticking to healthy diets on a regular basis. People who fast on a daily basis using the 16/8 method of intermittent fasting usually drop their total meals per day from three-plus to just two. This can be one meal in the morning and one in the evening. Some people eat snacks in between, but because the eating window isn't that long, there isn't a reason to snack that hard, especially if you take on a healthy, filling diet. Intermittent fasting is more of a lifestyle choice, which makes it easy for people to stick to a new dieting lifestyle for a longer time.

Fasting for Muscle Gain

Most studies on intermittent fasting have been done in regards to weight loss. If a person takes part in intermittent fasting without exercising, then weight loss will be a combination of both fat mass and lean mass. Lean mass includes everything, including muscle (excluding fat). This sort of lean-mass loss isn't only evident in intermittent fasting, but with other traditional diets as well. However, there have been a few studies that have shown that intermittent fasting does cause small amounts (around one kg/two pounds) of lean mass to be lost through consistently fasting for several months.

To confuse matters even further, other studies related to lean-mass loss have shown no loss when performing intermittent fasting. There are some researchers that believe that intermittent fasting is actually more effective at maintaining lean mass during weight loss when compared to non-fasting, calorie-restriction diets. However, as mentioned earlier, the research in this regard is still in its infancy, and more research is needed to prove this. In general, it is believed that intermittent fasting will not cause you to lose more muscle than any other diet will.

There is next to no research that promotes muscle gain when taking part in intermittent fasting. Probably one of the main reasons for this is that most studies focus more on the weight-loss aspect instead of muscle gain. That being said, there was one study that focused on intermittent fasting and weight training. Eighteen young men, who had never previously taken part in weight training, performed an eight-week weight training program.

The men in the study followed either a normal diet or a time-restricted diet, similar to intermittent fasting. The time-restricted diet required them to consume all their food within a daily four-hour window. At the end of the study, the group that practiced time-restricted eating had managed to maintain their lean body mass while increasing its strength. On the other hand, the group that ate a normal diet managed to gain lean mass (2.3 kg/five pounds) while also increasing its strength.

These results show that time-sensitive restrictive diets, similar to intermittent fasting, aren't necessarily the best in regards to muscle gain. One of the possible reasons for these results is that time-restricted eating means that the men were, in fact, consuming less protein than is needed for muscle gain. Another reason why the men with the restricted eating pattern were not able to gain muscle mass is that you need to consume more calories than you can burn, especially protein, to build muscle mass.

Intermittent fasting makes it difficult for you to consume the required amount of calories needed to build muscle, especially if your feasting window is very short and you consume low-carb meals that fill you up. This means that you will have to make a much larger effort to consume enough protein when you are eating less than usual. All being said, it doesn't necessarily mean that it is impossible to grow muscle mass while fasting. There still has to be a specific study aimed towards proving this first, before we know the actual results of muscle growth.

There has been research centered around weight training and how it can help prevent muscle loss when you are losing weight. There are a few studies that have shown muscle loss prevention in men who took part in intermittent fasting. An eight-week study, geared towards finding out the outcomes of intermittent fasting while weight training three days per week, split 34 men into two groups. The first group consumed calories only within an eight-hour window, while the other group was on a normal diet.

Both groups were allocated the same amount of calories and protein for daily consumption. The only real difference was the men with a shorter eating window. The study found that neither group lost strength or lean mass. The group that was on a time-restricted diet did, however, lose fat (1.6 kg/3.5 pounds). The group on the normal diet did not see any change. This study proves that weight training for three days per week actually helps to maintain muscle during fat loss as a result of intermittent fasting.

Another study was done on people who took part in alternate-day fasting while spending between 25 to 40 minutes on an exercise bike or elliptical trainer at least three times per week. These people maintained lean mass during weight loss. In general, if you wish to maintain muscle mass while fasting regularly, then it is advisable to perform regular exercise.

A popular question in regards to intermittent fasting and exercise is, should you exercise while fasting? Many debates have come as a result of this pressing question. Some people state that it is better to exercise while fasting, as your body isn't being bogged down by any sort of food or drink. Others argue that they need to eat something small, to have some kind of energy before they train.

One study placed 20 women on treadmills over a four-week period. Some of these women were fasting while exercising, while the other women performed non-fasted exercises. The participants in this study exercised for three days per week at one hour per session. The study found that both groups lost the same amount of weight and fat, with neither group having a change in lean mass. According to these results, it doesn't seem to matter if you exercise while you are fasting or not.

Nevertheless, people, in general, feel that training while fasting can impair your exercise performance, especially if you are a professional athlete. This is probably one of the reasons why most of the studies on intermittent fasting and weight training have not required subjects to exercise while they are fasting. If you do wish to train while fasting, you should be fine as long as you break your fast shortly afterward.

Fasting for Women

Intermittent fasting may affect women and men differently. There is evidence out there that states that intermittent fasting may not be as beneficial for some women as it is for men. One study found that blood sugar control worsens in women after three weeks of intermittent fasting. Such results were not the case in men. There has also been some talk centered around women who experience changes to their menstrual cycles once they begin intermittent fasting.

It is said that most of these sorts of shifts occur due to the extreme sensitivity of female bodies to calorie restriction. Fasting for long periods of time brings down a woman's calorie intake which affects their hypothalamus, a part of the brain. Such an event can disrupt the secretion of hormones, such as the gonadotropin-releasing hormone. This hormone also assists in releasing other hormones, such as the luteinizing hormone and the stimulating follicle hormone.

When these hormones are compromised in any such way, it makes it difficult for them to communicate with a woman's ovaries, which then results in irregular periods, poor bone health, infertility, and other related health conditions. At this moment there aren't any human-based studies available to prove that intermittent fasting can, without a doubt, cause adverse effects on women.

There have only been tests performed on lab animals, which have shown that alternate-day fasting for three to six months caused a reduction in ovary size as well as irregular reproductive cycles in female rats. It's best that woman take a more conservative, mild, and modified approach to intermittent fasting. Begin your intermittent fasting journey with shorter fasting windows and gradually extend your fasting times as your body similarly adapts to intermittent fasting.

Intermittent Fasting Benefits for Woman

Heart disease is among the leading causes of death worldwide. Some of the leading factors surrounding the development of heart disease are high blood pressure, cholesterol, and high triglyceride concentrations. One study found that women and men who took part in intermittent fasting managed to lower their blood pressure by six percent after eight weeks. The study also showed that intermittent fasting also reduced LDL cholesterol (by 25 percent) and triglycerides (by 32 percent).

It is important to note that no specific test or evidence fully links intermittent fasting with improved LDL cholesterol and triglyceride levels. There was a study that found no significant improvement in LDL cholesterol and triglycerides in women and men who undertook a 40-day intermittent fast during the month of Ramadan. People in general have reported improved heart health once they have begun fasting. However, there is no official evidence backed research or study out there that signifies the results that intermittent fasting has on a persons heart health. Official high-standard studies, with more capable testing methods, are needed to fully determine the effects of intermittent fasting on heart health.

It is possible that intermittent fasting can also effectively help manage the risk of diabetes. It is similar to how calorie consumption can help reduce some diabetic risk factors. A study that consisted of more than 100 overweight women found that intermittent fasting, over a period of six months, helped the women reduce insulin levels by 29 percent. The women also experienced a 19 percent reduction in insulin resistance, but their blood sugar levels remained the same.

Intermittent fasting may have its benefits, but it may not be as beneficial for women as it is for men. Another study found that blood sugar actually worsened for women after 22 days of intermittent fasting. This was through the alternate-day method of intermittent fasting. Despite this, it is still believed that the reduction in insulin resistance and insulin itself can still reduce the risk of diabetes, especially for individuals with pre-diabetes.

In regards to weight loss, there still aren't any effective weight-loss studies available that are specifically focused on women who perform intermittent fasts. Various studies and reports highlight the weight-loss experienced by adults in general over both short and long periods of time. The average weight loss of overweight adults after a year of intermittent fasting is seven kg (15 lbs). Short-term losses in body weight were around three to eight percent.

Best Methods of Intermittent Fasting for Women

As mentioned earlier, intermittent fasting for women is not a simple transition into a new style of eating. It is advised that women start fasting for smaller periods of time to allow their bodies time to adjust to their new eating habit. Women can also consume small amounts of calories on fast days, if they wish, before taking the leap into a full fast.

The different methods of intermittent fasting were discussed already, but there are a few adjusted methods that apply mainly to women.

Crescendo Method

Fast for 12 to 16 hours on either two or three days in a week. Any day is fine, as long as fasting days are not consecutive. An example would be to fast on Monday, Wednesday, and Friday. The best way to achieve a day's fast is not to eat anything in the evening and to skip your breakfast. If you have a late breakfast at 10 a.m., after your last meal at 6 p.m. the day before, then you can easily achieve 16 hours.

Eat-Stop-Eat – The 24-Hour Protocol

This is a full fast, at least once a week. It is also permissible to fast twice a week, if need be. Some people do push harder by fasting three times a week. This is not advised for women. The maximum number of days per week for women should be two days. It isn't necessary for women to fast the full 24-hour day. Just as with the crescendo method, women can start off with a 14- to 16-hour fast once a week.

However, fasting just once a week, for 14 hours, may be too less for you to adjust accordingly. The break from one fasting session to the next will be an entire week. This is far too long of a break for a person to settle into a decent rhythm. Try to advance to a larger fasting window as quickly as you can, or try out two days a week of fasting.

The 5:2 Diet

This is also called the "Fast Diet," which requires you to fast on two non-consecutive days. An example would be to fast on a Monday and Thursday. The fasts that you perform on these days allow you to consume around 500 calories. This can be one 500-calorie meal during each of your fasting days, or you could opt for two small 250-calorie meals. You are then allowed to eat normally, as you would on the other five non-fasting days.

Alternate-Day Fasting – Modified

Alternate-day fasting requires you to eat on one day, fast the next day, then eat again on the following day, and so on. You are required to fast for an entire day on your alternate-fast days and to eat normally on feast days. This is an excessive and advanced method and isn't usually advised for beginners or women in general. However, you can modify this fast to include about 500 calories on the days that you fast.

500 calories is about 25 percent of your normal daily intake and can either be had in one meal or split into two meals. This means that you will eat normally on one day, then restrict your intake to 500 calories the next day.

The 16/8 Method

The 16/8 method, also known as the Leangains method, consists of daily fasting for about 16 hours. This brings down your eating window to about eight hours. This is known as one of the easiest methods to adjust to as you fast daily, so implementing the fast in your daily life will be easy. Women are advised to begin this method on a shorter fasting window of 14 hours, to adjust to this method correctly.

If you choose to fast moderately by completing modified versions of intermittent fasts, then you should more or less be safe from any uncomfortable physical symptoms. There have been studies that have reported some side effects that groups of women have experienced while practicing intermittent fasting. Some of these side effects include mood swings, headaches, lack of concentration, and hunger on fasting days.

Apart from the studies, there have been complaints from women online who reported that their menstrual cycle stopped while they were on an intermittent fast. If you have moved from a moderate level to a more intense level of intermittent fasting and are beginning to experience uncomfortable symptoms, then you should move back to your moderate routine. Most of the symptoms can be overlooked, but if they get so bad that they actually make it difficult for you to work or carry out daily duties, then start toning it back a bit.

If you are someone who has a medical condition, then it is best to consult with a doctor first, before trying out intermittent fasting. Women who have had a history of eating disorders should consider this as well. Others that should receive a medical consultation before taking on intermittent fasting are:

- Women who are pregnant and breastfeeding

- Women who are trying to conceive

- Women who are underweight

- Women who have nutritional deficiencies

- Women who have diabetes

- Women who have low blood sugar levels

There hasn't been any serious medical condition that has come about as a result of intermittent fasting. Women should be safe, for the most part, when practicing intermittent fasting, especially if done moderately. If you do experience dramatic changes, such as loss of your menstrual cycle, then you should stop as soon as possible.

A Step-By-Step Guide to Intermittent Fasting

Step #1 – Consult a Doctor Before Starting an Intermittent Fast

It's best to seek out proper medical advice from your doctor before embarking on any diet. Intermittent fasting may have many health benefits, but it doesn't mean that you should overlook your own personal doctor's advice. It is possible that a doctor may advise against fasting if you have some form of the pre-existing medical condition.

Intermittent fasting can have a dramatic effect on your metabolism. Intermittent fasting can also affect a woman differently when compared to the effects it has on men. People who already have type 1 diabetes may not be able to handle long hours of fasting as they will have difficulty maintaining healthy insulin levels because they are not consuming food regularly enough to get their insulin going at a balanced rate.

Step #2 – Choose the Intermittent Fasting Method That Best Suits You

It's best to go with an intermittent-fasting method that will be easy to adopt and will suit your lifestyle. The 16/8 method, as well as the 5:2 method, are among the easiest to adopt and are considered beginner fasting methods. If you are looking for a lifestyle change, then the 16/8 is the way to go as it will require you to fast every day. This means that fasting will be a part of your daily life as you will need to implement it into your daily schedule and routines.

If you are not such an intense person but want to get into the world of intermittent fasting, then the 5:2 method is perfect, as it will require you to revisit your new fasting lifestyle for only two days in the week. Keeping up a weekly routine can definitely work, which is why the 5:2 method is an effective way of losing weight. You never know, you may enjoy this method so much that you might even begin to fast more on a regular basis.

The best method for absolute beginners who simply want a taste of intermittent fasting is the spontaneous meal-skipping method. This method gives you the flexibility to fast when you want. We are conditioned to make sure that we eat every single meal that is available to us. The spontaneous meal-skipping method allows us to skip meals from time to time, to get a taste of what fasting is with the hopes of also reaping some of the benefits.

Whatever method you choose, if you are inexperienced in fasting, it is advisable that you begin fasting for shorter periods than the methods require you to. Instead of fasting for 16 hours, try eight hours, and instead of going for a full day, do half-day fasts. Ease your way into fasting first, before you c begin to take on much more intense fasting sessions. Also make sure you drink enough water during your initial fasting sessions so that you remain hydrated throughout your fast.

Step #3 – Fast When You Are Asleep

One of the main reasons why the 16/8 method of intermittent fasting is so effective is that most of the time spent fasting is during the time you are asleep. When you sleep, your body obviously does not consume any food or unwanted calories. It also gives you the opportunity to fast for a short period while you are awake.

There are plenty of people that fast from sunrise to sunset. This means that these people have to wake up extra early to eat, then eat again in the evening. This sort of a routine actually breaks up your fasting times into shorter times, meaning that you are only allowing your body less time to burn fat. Try to fast for periods before and after you sleep. This way you can take advantage of your sleeping time without food.

Step #4 – Keep Track of Your Calories

Most diets require you to keep a close eye on your calorie intake. Intermittent fasting will automatically decrease your calorie intake as long as you usually eat during your eating window. However, it is easy to fall off the wagon when it is time to break your fast, especially if you are taking part in long, extended fasting periods. Counting your calories means that you will be aware of those moments when you unwillingly overeat.

If you are someone who always has, in some way or another, practiced healthy eating after doing some research, then you will already have an idea of the number of calories that are in your meals. If you are new to counting calories, then one of the quickest ways to get into counting calories is by using an app similar to MyFitnessPal or Lifesum. These are great apps that allow you to simply input the food that you are eating into the app.

The app will then calculate the calories for you. Some apps will even break down your daily calorie intake into macronutrients such as fat, protein, and carbs. This is ideal if you want to be on top of the exact nutrients that your body is receiving. However, you must be cautious as your exact calorie readings are usually just an estimate and should be seen as a guide. Calories differ due to the different brands of foods, and it is possible that you or the app could have made a calculation or input error.

Step #5 – Exercise

Exercise is recommended for all types of diets and weight-loss programs. Not only does working out help boost your weight-loss efforts, but it also promotes good health and longevity. This is why it is undoubtedly a great idea to exercise or to continue exercising while you begin your intermittent-fasting journey.

If you are a bit skeptical towards working out while you are fasting, then schedule your gym visits for a time that is within your eating window. An example would be to fast from 6 p.m. till 10 a.m. the next day (16-hour fast). You can then schedule your gym session for either 4 p.m. or 5 p.m., after work. This way you can have a few light snacks in the afternoon, before your gym session.

These snacks can help you to maintain good levels of energy before you get to the gym. Your last meal of the day can be right after you train, which will be ideal. You can also schedule your gym session for midday, when your energy levels are relatively high. Your meal at 10 a.m. should be sufficient to take you through to your workout. You can then snack on something afterward, like a post-workout protein snack.

There may come a time when you will want to workout in the morning while you are fasting. You can certainly do that, as long as it is not a high-intensity workout. A light run or cardio should be okay.

Chapter 3: Essentials of Eating

Scheduling Meals

When you begin your intermittent-fasting journey, you will be able to feel fuller for much longer. This will allow you the opportunity to keep your meals very simple. You can adjust your meals according to the intermittent-fasting method that you may choose. If you are planning on fasting for less than half a day, then you will be able to eat every meal of the day, including some additional snacks. An example would be to have an eating window from 8 a.m. to 6 p.m.

Once you have begun to ease into your fast, which mostly takes place in the evening, you can then slowly begin to extend your fasting hours. This is how most people who start with intermittent fasting begin to progress through to more advanced and longer fasts. Instead of fasting through the night and ending your fast at 8 a.m., try to push a little further, till about 10 a.m. This will give you a full 16-hour fast. Once you have mastered these times, you can then boost the time to 12 p.m.

If you only begin eating at 12 p.m. and stop eating at 6 p.m., then you will have narrowed your eating window to a mere six hours. This means that you will have to miss out on breakfast. If you are not a breakfast person, then this may be great news. However, there are plenty of people that insist that breakfast is their most important and favorite meal of the day. You can still eat the same meal at either 10 a.m. or 12 p.m., but you will have to skip out on lunch because you will already be full from your breakfast.

Not having lunch is not as difficult as you may think, as you will have had a late breakfast. After a few weeks of fasting this way, you will actually be fine with not having lunch because you will be feeling full, and waiting till dinner to eat won't be so bad. You can instead have an early dinner and begin your next fast. This will bring you to just two meals a day, which is perfect for those who wish to take part in intermittent fasting.

There's no problem with having snacks such as nuts and seeds in between your two meals for the day. You can even have another meal, if you like. However, it is best to limit your food and calorie intake during these times. You will naturally feel full during the midpoint of your eating window. As you progress on your intermittent-fasting journey, you will notice, as the weeks pass, that your entire mentality towards eating and food will change. You will begin to find a new love for food and will respect, conserve, and enjoy food in a whole new way.

The 5:2 method of fasting is another popular intermittent-fasting method. This is a suitable method for most people, as you only have to fast twice a week, meaning that there won't be much change to your current eating habits and routine. Just a whole-day sacrifice, twice a week. For the other five days, you will need to eat clean, meaning that you must try not to consume too much junk food on these days. It's best to stick to a healthy low-carb diet on these days.

On the days that you do fast, restrict yourself to 500 calories. If you are just starting this method of intermittent fasting, then it is advisable to consume 700 calories each day, until you are confident that you can go lower. Five-hundred calories is the sweet spot, as you can overcompensate at times because of calculation errors. One meal in the evening is fine, or you can break up the 500 calories into two small meals.

Popular advanced variations of the 5:2 plan don't allow you to eat anything during the two nonconsecutive days of the week. If you choose Monday and Thursday as your two fasting days, then you will be prohibited from eating anything on these two days. No food at all from the time you wake up till you go to bed, then clean eating for the rest of the five days. This may sound excessive, but it is entirely achievable, especially if you keep up with water consumption.

For those who are really into intermittent fasting and have mastered many methods of fasting, there is an advanced every-other-day plan which allows you eat on one day then do a full complete fast the next day, with no food at all, and to eat normally the following day. This is an excessive method of intermittent fasting, as you will have full days without food every alternate day. Those who have undertaken this method of fasting say this method produced excellent results.

When it is time to eat, you should try and stick to healthy fats, clean meat, and vegetables, with some fruit. On your full-fasting days, it's just water. With the option for black tea or coffee. You can also sip on some herbal tea if you like, as long as there is no sugar or milk. As mentioned earlier, mindset plays a huge role when fasting. As you advance into fasting and start getting better at it, fasting an entire day can become second-nature for you.

Use an app such as MyFitnessPal or Lifesum to track your meals. These apps give you proper breakdowns of your meals in regards to calories, fat, carbs, and protein. The Fitbit app also has an excellent food-tracking feature. Once you have come to understand how much calories are in the food that you are eating, you will then be able to simply pick out the right food to eat at the right times.

Intermittent Fasting and the Ketogenic Diet

The state at which your body switches over from its primary energy source in glucose (derived from carbs) to an alternate energy source in ketones (derived from fats) is known as ketosis. Once you have achieved a state of ketosis, your body will then rely on fats for energy. This means that you will turn your body into a fat-burning machine. To achieve this, you will have to cut out the carbs that are usually used to fuel your body.

There are two ways in which you can heavily restrict your carb intake. One way is to fast regularly, and the other way is to take on a low-carb diet such as the ketogenic diet. The ketogenic diet (keto diet) is an extremely low-carb, medium-to low-protein, high-fat diet. Practicing this diet in tandem with intermittent fasting means that you can allow your body's glucose reserve to deplete fully. In doing so, your body will then begin to start converting fat into ketones for energy.

Relying only on intermittent fasting to achieve a fat-burning state of ketosis isn't so simple. Your body needs time to switch over into ketosis, which is usually about two to seven days. Fasting regularly, while consuming plenty of carbs during your eating window, won't allow you to remain in a ketosis state. You will have to adjust your diet accordingly to remove unwanted carbs. The keto diet is the way to go if you wish to achieve this.

What is the Keto Diet?

The keto diet, short for the ketogenic diet, is a low-carb, high-fat diet. The purpose of this diet is to restrict carbs to a bare minimum to promote ketosis, a fat-burning state that uses ketones derived from fat, either from your body's fat stores or from the food you eat. This is why the keto diet consists of up to 75 percent of fat consumption. The calorie breakdown looks something like this:

- 60 - 75% fat

- 15 - 30% protein

- 5 - 10% carbs

The keto diet does allow for protein, but at a controlled and reduced amount. Consuming too much protein can cause the excess protein that you consume to be converted into glucose. This can disturb the process of ketosis. The keto diet relies on the fats that you consume for energy. Your body will process these fats into ketones which can be used to fuel your body and brain. If you carefully follow the keto diet eating plan, then your body will transition over into ketosis, which usually takes about two to seven days.

How Does Ketosis Work?

As mentioned before, the physical state of ketosis usually arises when your body doesn't have any carbs to feed your cells to produce energy. As a solution for this, your body will begin to generate ketones, organic compounds that your body then uses in place of the missing carbs. So instead of your body shutting down due to a low carb/glucose energy source, it will, in a smart way, turn to fat/ketones. When this happens, your body will have to burn fat faster than usual so that it can consistently generate the appropriate amount of ketones.

Ketones can be seen as an alternative fuel for your body, which, on a regular basis, relies only on carbs which are broken down into blood sugar or glucose. When your body is in short supply of glucose, it will then look to an alternate energy source such as ketones. This is the main reason that the keto diet only allows for an extremely low amount of carbs so that you can force your body to begin working towards using its alternate energy source.

Your body and your brain rely on either glucose or ketones as an energy source and not simply carbs or fat itself. Whether it's carbs or fats, your body will break down whatever food you eat into molecules which can then be used as energy. So if you successfully practice the keto diet, you will be able to force your body to switch its fuel supply to run entirely on fat, which is further broken down into molecules known as ketones. The reason the switch over to a ketosis state takes a few days is that your body is busy finishing off its carb/glucose reserve.

When achieving a ketosis state, your body's insulin levels will be low. As a result, it will be easier than ever for your body to access the stored energy (fat stores) to burn them off. Achieving this is perfect for those who are looking to lose weight. Another benefit behind this is having a steady supply of energy, which can also assist you in regulating hunger.

Types of Keto Diets

There are a few different types of keto diets, each designed to suit people from all different kinds of backgrounds with different lifestyles. Because of this, it can be easy for you to transition into the keto diet. Some versions of the keto diet actually allow you to consume carbs as well. These versions are great, especially if you are an athlete or bodybuilder. These modified and targeted diets are seen as advanced versions of the keto diet and are best suited for those professional athletes that may adopt them.

Standard Ketogenic Diet – SKD

This is the standard version of the keto diet that everyone knows about. This version consists of a very low carb intake, with moderate protein and high fat. Your calorie consumption should look like this: five percent carbs, 20 percent protein, 75 percent fat.

High-Protein Ketogenic Diet

The high-protein ketogenic diet is very similar to the standard ketogenic diet. In this diet, you just adjust your protein intake from 20 percent to 35 percent, while keeping your carb intake to a minimum. Your calorie consumption should look like this: five percent carbs, 35 percent protein, 60 percent fat.

Cyclical Ketogenic Diet – CKD

This diet allows for higher carb refeeds during some periods. Carb refeeds meaning meals that allow for a higher percentage of carbs (about 250 grams of carbs compared to the current diets 50 grams). The keto diet only allows for 5% of carbs. This means that your body will go for a long time without carbs. A short carb refeed can restore some balance to a diet based on prolonged carb restriction. An example of this would be to follow the keto diet correctly for five days of the week while consuming carbs for the remaining two days of the week.

Targeted Ketogenic Diet

This version of the keto diet allows you to consume carbs around the time when you perform your workouts or physical activities.

The most recommended diets from this list are the standard keto diet and the high-protein keto diet. Apart from all of the benefits of these two diets, they are, in fact, the most researched diets on the list, as the rest of the diets are advanced modified variants of the keto diet. There has not been that much research conducted on the cyclical and targeted keto diets.

Research has shown that the keto diet is much more effective in losing weight when compared to other low-fat diets. One of the reasons for this is that the keto diet is a high-fat intake diet. Consuming food that is high in fat will naturally leave you feeling less hungry later on. The same cannot be said for other calorie-restriction diets which, in most cases, leave people hungry as they continuously count calories. On a keto diet, it is still possible to lose weight even without restricting one's calorie intake.

One study, in particular, showed that people on the keto diet were able to lose more than two times the weight of those other people who were on a low-fat diet. The same study showed that the participants' HDL cholesterol and triglyceride levels also improved. The keto diet allows your body to remain in ketosis. This means that your body's increased levels of ketones will assist in lowering your blood sugar levels while improving insulin sensitivity. These beneficial factors of a keto diet are among the reasons behind the diet's ability to help people lose weight efficiently while living a healthy lifestyle.

Exercising While You Are Fasting

Those of us who love spending time in the gym also love spending equal amounts of time in the kitchen. Eating healthy meals all the time is more or less a part of living healthy and keeping healthy. Intermittent fasting isn't necessarily an end to any of these. You can still enjoy great food and exercise on a regular difference. The only major difference is that you will not be able to eat during specified eating windows.

So how does this affect your workout regime? Are you someone who has to have a pre-workout shot before you enter the gym? Do you need a blast of protein right after the gym? Can you still build muscle if you train while you fast?

When you are physically active, your body mainly uses glycogen, which is stored carbohydrates, as fuel for exercise. The only exception to this is when your glycogen reserves have been fully depleted. This is possible if you haven't eaten in a while. So, with the exception of not having any glycogen fuel, your body will seek out alternative energy sources in the form of fat. The *British Journal of Nutrition* posted a study which had men run before eating breakfast. These men managed to burn up 20 percent more fat than men who ate breakfast before they ran.

Your body also has the potential to break down protein when

in short supply of glycogen. This means that intermittent fasting will cause you to lose fat as well as muscle when you workout and fast. If you decide to go out on a run while fasting, chances are your body will begin to burn protein. Working out while fasting can also possibly slow down your metabolism, which can have an effect on how you lose weight in the long run. When you workout, your body will require more calories. But if you are fasting, then your body will have to adapt to fewer calories, which means a slower metabolism.

It's important to be careful when looking up advice regarding physical training while fasting. There are mixed feelings towards this exact subject as there has not been any solid proof of the actual muscle gains or losses from working out while fasting. Similar studies were done in which men who trained while fasting didn't lose any muscle mass or lean mass. Instead, they maintained their lean mass and only lost body fat.

However, the problem with most of these studies is that these men usually eat right after working out. There still has to be a study that analyzes men who workout while they fast without them eating anything after the workout. There also has to be a study with the effects of pre-workout and post-workout supplements with men who workout while they are fasting.

Tips on Working Out While Fasting

Working out is definitely recommended for those who practice intermittent fasting as workouts can help boost weight loss. However, it's best to workout within an eating window, just to be safe. Some people may find cardio workouts great during periods while they are fasting. This is okay as long as you try to eat something shortly after you have trained.

So, no need to throw in the towel, keep going with your workouts. Working out regularly is just as important to your health as intermittent fasting is, both physically and mentally. Here are a few tips on planning your workouts in order to get the most out of them while fasting.

Tip #1 Cardio Intensity

It's best to keep your cardio intensity low if you are fasting while you workout. Keep track of your breathing as this can be a good clue on how far your body can go while fasting. It can be easy to get carried away and overdo your cardio effort levels as your body is light from no food, making it easier to accomplish your cardio routines. This is why you should pay attention to your breathing.

You should be okay if you plan on going for a small walk or jog while fasting or even a low-effort elliptical session. Stop exercising if you feel lightheaded or dizzy while you are working out. This could be your body warning you to stop. We like to push past these symptoms in order to gain the next level of fitness. Just don't overdo the intensity or duration of your workout if you feel this way while fasting.

Tip #2 Go High Intensity Once You Have Broken Your Fast

There certainly isn't anything wrong with light exercise while fasting, especially if you keep yourself well hydrated. However, you shouldn't try high-intensity workouts during your fasting window, as mentioned above. You can step things up when you are working out during your eating window.

Some intermittent-fasting programs, such as the Leangains program, advise you to schedule meals around your workouts in order to maximize fat loss while still staying fueled up.

The closer you schedule moderate to intense workout sessions to your last meal, the better. This way, you will be able to have some leftover carbs, in the form of glycogen, to help fuel your workout. Consider snacking on some light carbs after an intense workout so that you can feed your glycogen-tapped muscles.

Tip #3 Eat High-Protein Meals

Regardless of whether you are fasting or not, you will need to consume decent amounts of protein if you wish to build muscle. As mentioned earlier, your body can drain its glucose, fat, and even protein reserves when you are fasting and working out. This is why it makes sense to stock up on protein, to compensate for any protein loss from fasting. You can also create some outstanding muscle mass while you are at it.

A pre-workout snack may just be a good idea, especially if you are fasting. Yes, you are not allowed to eat anything while you fast, but you are about to embark on a gym session while on an empty stomach. Check the ingredients of your pre-workout snack or drink before you have it. If it has carbs that are less than 50 calories, then you should be okay to consume such a supplement while you are fasting.

While you fast, it is okay to consume a total of 50 calories. However, this should only really be made up of beverages such as coffee or tea. You can substitute these with small amounts of supplements when you fast. Just don't overdo it and go above the 50-calorie mark. When in your eating window, try to consume between 20 to 30 grams of high-quality protein, especially after training.

If you want to take your workout to the next level, then try and schedule your workouts between the two meals within your eating window while ensuring you consume the right amount of protein in these meals.

Tip #4 Keep on Snacking

If you do schedule your workout during your eating window, then you can even schedule snacks about three to four hours before your workout. Intermittent fasting promotes small snacks between meals. Having a healthy, simple snack that has fast-acting carbs, with blood sugar stabilizing protein, a few hours before you workout can give you a good blast of energy once it is time to workout. No junk food though!

Try to complement your workout by chowing down on a post-workout snack that contains around 20 grams of protein as well as 20 grams of carbs. Such a snack promotes muscle growth and can assist your body in finding its glycogen stores. These simple snacks can help you to remain energized.

Types of Foods for Intermittent Fasting

It is always important to remember that, when changing your diet for a diet that you have never done before, it is best to consult with a GP or health professional first before you make your decision. This doesn't just apply to the type of food that you will eat while fasting, but to any lifestyle diet change. Your body has to adapt to the change in nutrients that it will be receiving and if you have a medical condition, then that adaptation may not be as simple as you may think.

That being said, when it comes to intermittent fasting, the restrictions that you will face are mostly placed on when to eat rather than on what you can eat. Intermittent fasting isn't, in fact, a diet, but more of a lifestyle choice that assists you in cutting down on your calorie intake by decreasing your daily eating window. This means that you can still eat whatever you want during those eating windows. However, the question is, should you eat whatever you want?

Consuming too many varieties of junk food during your eating window will boost your overall calorie intake. Having chocolate and ice cream in the afternoon, after a good period of fasting, does sound tempting, especially after a long hard day of fasting. However, you will be wasting your fasting efforts as the junk food you consume will compensate for the calories that you missed out on. Moreover, when you feel sated from the junk food, that means the opportunity to for the body to replenish its required minerals and vitamins from nutrient-dense natural foods will be gone. It's best to work towards maintaining a well-balanced and healthy diet while fasting.

A proper, healthy diet can help you to maintain energy levels throughout the day and is also key to losing weight. The focus should be on nutrient-dense food such as vegetables, fruits, nuts, beans, seeds, whole grains, beans, dairy, and lean proteins. If you are known for eating an unhealthy diet, then try to switch things up by looking for food that can assist with improved health such as food that is high in fiber, whole foods, and even unprocessed food. These kinds of foods are good for your health and also help you stay full after you eat. Here are a few examples of these healthy types of food.

Fish

Most dietary guidelines recommend that you consume at least eight ounces of fish per week. In doing so, you will be providing yourself with generous amounts of vitamin D as well as healthy fats and protein. Fish can also be considered good for your cognitive function and is labeled as brain food by many people.

Avocados

Avocados are considered to be among the highest calorie fruits. For that reason, avocados may not be a good choice for those trying to watch their weight, but the fruit does have a decent amount of monounsaturated fat. This is part of the reason why avocados are very satiating to eat. Adding half an avocado to your lunch can assist in keeping you feeling full for hours longer than other fruits or vegetables.

Potatoes

Not all white foods are as bad as you think. Just like avocados, potatoes are among the most satiating foods available. There are studies that prove that eating potatoes as part of a healthy diet can, in fact, aid with weight loss. One fact, in particular, is that when potatoes are cooked in healthy ways, they actually won't cause any harm to weight-loss plans. Some examples of healthy methods of cooking potatoes are baking them, boiling, steaming, and roasting. Potatoes are known to be complex carbohydrates and can aid in weight loss.

Eggs

Eggs are considered an excellent source of protein and are easy and quick to cook. One medium- to large-sized egg has about six grams of protein. Consuming protein is a great way to build muscle. One study, in particular, found that men who ate eggs for breakfast over a bagel were less hungry after breakfast. These men also ate less throughout the day. There are more current studies aimed towards the benefits of eating eggs and also toward debunking the idea that eggs are harmful because of cholesterol.

Whole Grains

Eating carbs while on a diet isn't always a bad thing, especially if you consume whole grains that are rich in fiber and protein. Eating just a little will go a long way in keeping you full. One study, in particular, found that eating whole grains instead of refined grains may actually assist in increasing your metabolism. Experiment with different types of whole grains such as bulgur, kamut, and amaranth.

Nuts

Nuts are known to have more calories than most snacks. However, nuts contain healthy fats that are good for your body. Studies show that polyunsaturated fat in walnuts can alter the physiological markers that are related to satiety and hunger. Nuts are also known to carry some key benefits like the ability to reduce metabolic syndrome risk factors such as cholesterol levels and high blood pressure.

Berries

All types of berries are known to contain crucial nutrients. Strawberries are an excellent source of immune-boosting vitamin C. Studies have shown that people who consume food that is rich in flavonoids, such as blueberries, have smaller increases in their BMI over a 14-year period than those who do not eat berries. The bottom line is that berries are good for you for many reasons such as being low in carbs yet high in fiber and antioxidants. Most berries have proven benefits towards heart health as well.

Beans and Legumes

It is known that food such as chickpeas, black beans, peas, and lentils can assist in decreasing body weight without calorie restriction. Beans and legumes may consist of carbs, but they are low-calorie carbs which won't hurt your eating plan. These are the sort of carbs that can assist in supplying you with energy, without all the excess calories.

Cruciferous Vegetables

Food such as broccoli, cauliflower, and Brussels sprouts are filled with fiber. These are also the kinds of foods that can help keep you regular by assisting in preventing constipation. Food with fiber can also make you feel full. This is especially useful if you intend to go without food for a while due to fasting.

Fluids Allowed When Fasting

Most people who take part in intermittent fasting consume water while they fast. Consuming water is prohibited when undergoing certain religious fasts. However, that isn't the case with intermittent fasting as it is advised that you stay hydrated with water while you fast, as long as it is only water that you consume while fasting, and not food. Not consuming water may cause you to become dehydrated which can result in headaches and general fatigue. You don't want to be experiencing this while you have not eaten.

If you are undertaking a 16-hour fast, then not drinking any water will not get you into any trouble as far as dehydration is concerned. The chances of you becoming dehydrated depend on many factors, such as the weather and your behavior, and whether you are active or not. If you have a decent amount of water during the evening before you start fasting, then you should be okay the next day.

Apart from water, the only other beverages that are acceptable are coffee or tea. Drinking these hot beverages is acceptable while fasting as they do not have that many calories in them and will not genuinely affect your weight-loss efforts. Unfortunately, you cannot add any other ingredients to your coffee or tea while you are fasting. This means no cream, sugar, or milk. These items contain added calories that you should stay away from when you are fasting. It is a massive no to other beverages such as soda and juices.

Chapter 4: Getting Around Speed Bumps

The Common Mistakes of Intermittent Fasting and How to Avoid Them

#1: Eating Junk Food

When you initially start fasting, you will most likely find yourself counting down the minutes until you're allowed to eat again. As a result, your mind will cause you to develop cravings for things that you like to eat because they taste good and will satisfy you, i.e., junk foods such as chocolate, potato chips, and fizzy drinks, to name a few. It's natural for your body to crave what it's being denied, but this is where an element of self-control is needed, as well as a basic understanding of the concept of intermittent fasting.

When you fast, your body becomes an efficient, self-cleaning machine. It breaks down not only fats but also its damaged components and converts them to energy. This process cleans and repairs the entire body, promoting it to work as efficiently as possible for optimum health. Hence, what you put into your body is of great importance.

To achieve the best results from intermittent fasting, you have to try and consume foods that are high in nutrients and low in fat and sugar. Nutrient-rich foods will provide your body with the nourishment it needs, especially in the fasted state, and also will keep you fuller for longer. Even though you are eating fewer meals a day, filling up those meals with junk food will only lead you towards more unhealthy food cravings. This is because junk food doesn't provide your body with the nourishment it needs and will cause you to feel hungry again more quickly. This can only lead you to cheat by breaking your fast.

What Steps Can You Take to Avoid Giving in to Junk Food Cravings?

The digital age is a complete blessing in this instance as there are quite a few calorie-counting apps now available to help you track your intake every time you eat a meal. These apps can be most useful by giving you an idea of how many calories you are consuming per meal item, so you will be able to make better choices when deciding what to eat, and how much to eat, i.e., portion size.

Another useful tip is meal prep. Preparing your meals ahead of time can save you the frustration that comes from fasting and being hungry, and thus can save you from giving in to your cravings. By having a meal ready, you don't have to go through that sometimes arduous and time-consuming process of cooking a meal after an extended period of fasting. This frustration can lead you to binge on junk food while you're cooking and this can lead you to go over your maximum calorie intake before you've ever eaten your meal.

Lastly, I would advise you to indulge your body and give in to those cravings, but only after you have eaten a proper, nutrient-rich meal. Your hunger will be sated, and therefore you will be less likely to overindulge.

Even though intermittent fasting works best because you eat

less, it doesn't mean that you can eat what you want. Nutrient-rich all the way!

#2: Over-Restricting Calorie-Intake

A big concern when you are trying out the intermittent-fasting method is not eating enough food during the eating window. Sometimes people can go overboard and start over-restricting their calorie intake because they feel this will help them lose weight faster. This is completely untrue. When you don't consume enough calories per day, your body goes into emergency mode. So instead of using your body's fat stores to create energy, it stores the fat for use in the future and proceeds to feed on its own muscle mass. This will, in turn, cause your metabolism to slow down, which is the complete opposite of what you want.

A slower metabolism means you will lose weight at a very slow pace or sometimes not at all, and your fast will be for naught. Frequently, a slower metabolism can cause other adverse or undesirable effects on your body and will not be good for you in the long term. Signs include dry and cracked heels, hair loss, fat storage in places you've never noticed before, and sugar cravings, to name a few.

So the important thing to remember when trying out the intermittent-fasting method is to eat enough food during your eating window. You need to listen to your body and feed your metabolism to lose weight. The trick is to listen to your body and to feed it the right kind of foods that will promote an increased metabolic rate.

How Do I Make Sure I Am Eating Enough?

Once again, you can make use of those calorie-counting apps so that you can determine how much to eat for each meal, and make sure you're meeting your daily quota of calories, and therefore, energy.

Another idea is to consult a dietician. Although this might not be an option for those wishing to save money, it has the added benefit of professional advice based on you and your body specifically. A dietician will be able to tell you what foods will be good for you according to your blood type and body mass index, and will take into consideration any comorbidities you might suffer from.

If you're not one for gadgets and gizmos, scales and measuring cups, and you want to make intermittent fasting work for you in the simplest way possible, all you need are your hands. This guideline works as such:

- The size of your palm determines the size of your protein portion.

- The side of your fist determines your veggie portion.

- The size of your cupped hand determines your carb portion.

- The size of your thumb determines your fat portion.

If you're a man, it is recommended that you use two times the allotted portion size per protein, veggie, carb, and fat. If you're a woman, one portion size for each is recommended. Even though intermittent fasting works best because you eat less, it doesn't mean that you should eat as little as possible.

Remember to listen to your body.

#3: Eating Too Much During the Eating Window

A common trap that many people fall into when they start the intermittent-fasting method is that they overeat when they break their fast. They may be eating all the right foods, rich in nutrients, but they are eating way too much. This can occur because we all have some kind of emotional attachment to food; for some of us, it may be a bit more pronounced than others.

We've all heard the adage that some people eat to live, while others live to eat. Some of us use food to deal with our emotions and how fulfilled we feel in our lives. For example, you'll find newly-wedded couples indulging in dinners of pasta and wine more than once a week because they're all happy and in love. And how many of us have taken to polishing off a whole tub of ice-cream after a bad breakup?

So because you're depriving your body of food, the very thing that sustains it, your emotional state can dip very low, and in an effort to uplift your spirits, you can go overboard and binge. The primary focus of the intermittent fast is to listen to your body. Your body is designed to tell you when to stop eating, and it does this by releasing hormones to make you feel full or sated.

How Can I Avoid Overeating?

The aforementioned method of using your hands to gauge appropriate portion sizes for each food type will work really well here. You can once again make use of the calorie-counting apps and dietician visits for professional guidelines.

Another thing you can do is prepare something you really like to eat for each meal, keeping in mind that it is not high in fat or sugar. This is to ensure that not only will you be eating the right kind of foods but that you will also enjoy your meal. Sating both your physical and emotional hunger will leave you feeling more fulfilled and less likely to develop cravings. Win-win!

#4: Not Drinking Enough Water

The intermittent-fasting regimen will cause a decrease in the amount of hydration you would normally get from eating fruits and vegetables. Therefore you should make an extra effort to drink more than the recommended daily eight glasses of water a day. If you don't, your body will go into a dehydrated state, in addition to already being in the fasted state. This can lead to headaches and unclear thinking, muscle cramps, constipation, kidney stones, and even cause an increase in hunger pangs and junk-food cravings. You will be able to survive with no water for 16 hours. However, it is not advised to do this that often. It's best to stay hydrated.

When your body is in the fasted state, it starts to break down damaged components and toxins, and water is essential for these processes to flush them out of your system. It is recommended to drink approximately 11 cups of water for women, and 16 cups of water for men each day. The Centers for Disease Control and Prevention recommend "letting your thirst be your guide" as a way to stay hydrated. Not only will drinking more water keep you hydrated, but it will keep you fuller for longer by helping to stave off those hunger pangs.

How Can I Include More Water Intake Daily?

You can try to drink a full glass of water before and after each time you eat a meal in your eating window. You can also stay hydrated by including more water-based soups or broths in your eating window. These are not only satisfying to the soul but are also good low-calorie options. While you are fasting, you can motivate yourself to drink more and more water when you would normally have a meal. You can use the clock to set targets for water consumption, or in between completing your daily tasks at work or home.

You can also stay hydrated by drinking tea or coffee, but to keep the calories down, these have to be black. No milk, cream, or sugar! Artificial sweeteners can be used but in moderation. You can also try fruit-infused water to keep things exciting and satisfy your taste buds. Many people opt for strawberries or lemon, but tastes and combinations vary.

#5: Obsessing Over the Clock

In the beginning, the intermittent-fasting method may be harder for some and can lead to obsessing over the clock. The stress of this new change on your body, combined with the inevitable hunger, will leave you counting down the minutes and seconds until you can finally eat again.

How Do I Stop Obsessing?

If you want to stay true to your fast and have it work best for your body, it's important to occupy your mind by engaging fully in your work or daily tasks. You can even use the time to set new goals for yourself to accomplish each day to help divert your attention away from the hunger. You can try to fill up your time by doing things you find enjoyable such as reading or catching up on a TV show.

Any pleasurable activity that will keep you busy is recommended so that you will not be emotionally starved as you are physically starved. This will also associate the fasting with pleasurable activities, which helps with overall motivation. Take all this newfound time to accomplish something you've always wanted to do but have never done, or use the time to do things you usually don't have time for, like walking your dog or starting that organic garden you always wanted. Take the time to feed your soul!

Frequently Asked Questions

Which is the best type of intermittent fasting?

The best type of intermittent fasting that is agreed upon by the majority of the fitness and dietary worlds is the 16/8 Method or the Leangains Protocol.

Why?

- The main reason is that it is a type of fasting that you can implement every day, without any "cheat days," and it therefore has the greatest potential of becoming a permanent lifestyle.

- It allows your body to utilize your fat stores for energy consumption on a daily basis during the fasting hours when food is unavailable. This results in losing weight at a steady daily pace and therefore is a more sustainable form of weight loss.

- It is also easier to maintain because it incorporates your sleeping time into the 16-hour fast. This means that you will not be subjected to hunger pangs while you are asleep. And you can choose your eight-hour eating window to suit yourself. For example, if you are someone who needs to start the day with breakfast, you can set your eating window from 8 a.m. to 6 p.m. Or if you feel you can skip breakfast altogether, you can choose to eat between 11 a.m. and 7 p.m., giving you enough time to prepare dinner after getting home from work.

How can I prepare myself for intermittent fasting?

- Do your research properly. You're already off to a great start by reading this book but you can also find out more from people all over the web, which will give you a wider understanding of the concept as a whole.

- Consult your doctor on whether this option is suitable for you. Fasting and subsequent hunger pangs can cause a lot of stress and therefore may not be the best option for people already suffering from stress and anxiety disorders, especially those suffering from eating disorders. It can also be dangerous in type 1 diabetics, patients suffering from stomach and intestinal problems, and those with clinical myopathy (muscle- wasting disease).

- Pick an eating window that suits you best. As mentioned before, the eating window can be tailored to suit your specific lifestyle so try and choose one that will be easiest to maintain for you personally.

- Get into the habit of consuming more water. As mentioned previously, approximately 11 cups of water a day should suffice if you are a woman; and if you are a man, around 16 cups a day should do it.

- Make a list of things you can do to fill up the time and keep your mind busy while you are fasting. This can be a fun activity which will allow you to set goals you previously wouldn't have thought about.

- Take a picture of yourself before you start fasting so you can determine if this is working for you and to monitor your progress. This can also have the added benefit of keeping you motivated to stay on track.

How and what should I eat during the eating window?

The eating window is not meant for you to cram as much as you can during that time. And while it's important to eat the foods you love, you have to exercise caution and make sure you're not overindulging in things that are deemed unhealthy. Try to eat balanced meals that are rich in nutrients and which have components that you like in particular. Strive to incorporate lean proteins, fruits and vegetables, eggs and dairy, and healthy fats into your diet so that you have a variety of nutrients from different sources and a variety of meal options so things don't get boring.

For example, if your feeding window is from 10 a.m. to 6 p.m., you can use liquids like tea, coffee, or fruit-infused water to keep yourself full until 10 a.m. At that point, you can choose to have a proper breakfast and a lighter meal for lunch, or a small meal to keep you full until lunchtime so that your main meals are lunch and supper. Others choose to have a good meal for supper and resume drinking liquids after the feeding window closes, which in this case is at 6 p.m. You can choose what works for you.

What is a circadian rhythm and how does it relate to intermittent fasting?

A circadian rhythm can be defined as the physical, mental, and behavioral changes that occur in living beings over a daily cycle, i.e., a 24-hour period. They are built-in cycles that respond to an organism's exposure to external sources such as light and temperature. For example, we have a built-in circadian rhythm of sleeping patterns that respond to light in that we sleep at night and are awake during the day.

So, with regards to intermittent fasting, it is a frequently mentioned term because most research supports the use of our body's circadian rhythms, i.e., sleep-wake cycles when planning your fasting schedule. There also exists a circadian rhythm to hunger which can be tracked by the hunger hormone ghrelin. Research has shown that ghrelin is lowest in the mornings when you wake. So, contrary to popular belief, we are not the hungriest in the mornings and therefore do not need to start the day with a large breakfast. Ghrelin levels typically peak at around 1 to 2 p.m. and begin to dip again afterward towards the evening. This suggests that the day-and-night cycle also affects hunger, in that we are hungrier during daylight hours.

So by choosing to schedule your eating window with your body's circadian day-and-night cycle-related rhythms, the 10 a.m. to 6 p.m. feeding period can work best here where you focus on the main meal at around lunchtime and a smaller meal at dinnertime. The key to intermittent fasting has always been about listening to your body, and in this way, you are listening and responding to your ghrelin (hunger hormone) levels and are thus feeding your body accordingly.

Will intermittent fasting cause me to lose muscle mass?

In the fitness community, it's a common belief that intermittent fasting leads to muscle loss. When you lose weight by any method, it's important to remember that you lose both lean mass and fat mass. This is true for intermittent fasting as well as other diets. Studies have shown that you don't lose any more muscle mass when intermittent fasting as compared to being on any other weight-loss diets.

Is it true, however, that intermittent fasting may not be the best way to gain muscle mass if that is your primary goal. Because of the smaller amount of calories consumed with the intermittent- fasting regime, your body won't be getting enough calories, and in particular, protein to help you build muscle.

Can I workout when I am intermittent fasting?

Yes, you can do this. If you want to maintain your muscle mass as you lose weight, studies prove that weight-training is recommended to help you do this.

Should I workout when I am intermittent fasting?

Within the intermittent-fasting community, there is great debate about whether you should exercise when you are intermittent fasting if weight loss is your primary goal. Studies conducted to determine if weight loss is greater when exercising when fasting, as opposed to when not fasting, show that weight loss results are ultimately the same.

So it all boils down to what you prefer. Many people choose to workout because they enjoy it and because they want to maintain their body's muscle mass, as mentioned above. Others opt to not exercise in the fasted state because it can sometimes decrease levels of endurance and performance.

How can I include my working-out time when intermittent fasting?

The best way you can achieve this is actually to plan your meals around your workouts. So if you have chosen the 16/8 method, as recommended above, you should plan to exercise in the morning, before your eating window commences.

Cardio is best done on an empty stomach, so morning runs or spin classes are a great option. However, if you know that you will be working out the next day, it's advisable to make sure you have enough available energy to do so. You can do this by eating enough complex carbs for your last meal the day before. It's essential to plan ahead, to make sure that your body has enough nutrients and energy for the demands of the intensity of the workout.

With this in mind, it's also important to not pick a high-intensity workout for the morning because this is at the end of your fasting period, where energy stores are at a low. So if you are working out intensely, without the energy reserve to back it up, you may feel lightheaded and could actually pass out.

Cardio is not the greatest option when you have just eaten a meal because your muscles will demand most of your blood flow; blood flow that is needed for digesting and absorbing what you ate. As a result, you can end up feeling very bloated or nauseous, and may become sick.

So the key is to plan ahead: try to incorporate more complex carbs into your eating window when you know will be working out. For those days that you choose to take a rest, you can opt to fill your meals with more proteins, fats, and fruits and vegetables.

Is it safe to intermittent fast if I am pregnant?

There hasn't been enough research to determine if intermittent fasting is harmful when pregnant because it's unethical to put pregnant women on a diet (of any kind) for research purposes.

When you are pregnant, you certainly are eating for two, so naturally, your body's demand for nutritional value will be much greater. And it's important to meet those demands to ensure the healthy development of your baby. As a result, intermittent fasting should be avoided when pregnant.

Why do I get headaches when I intermittent fast?

When you first start intermittent fasting, your body can have some trouble adapting to this new schedule and lower calorie intake and therefore, many in the initial stages complain about headaches.

When you fast, your blood sugar levels take a dive and the first organ to feel this is the brain. The added elements of dehydration and increased stress hormones when you fast can also contribute to this. So try to drink as much water as you can by sticking to the aforementioned guideline of 11 cups for women and 16 cups for men per day. You can also try to incorporate liquids into your meal options like soups, and broths, to keep hydrated for longer. After a few days, the headaches will disappear.

I was told that intermittent fasting improves brain function, so why do I feel mentally sluggish?

In the initial stages of intermittent fasting, the brain has to adjust to all the changes mentioned above and therefore you may feel as though you are more sluggish in your thought processes. This will pass as the days go by and you will experience an increase in our brain function.

Is intermittent fasting a long-term solution for weight loss?

Yes, because it's not a diet in the typical sense of the word, but rather a lifestyle choice. And it has the whole host of added benefits mentioned previously that will make your lifestyle choice a healthier and more fulfilling one, leading you to feel better about yourself in all respects. Even if you do have a very unhealthy diet, intermittent fasting will still be able to automatically cut down on your overall calorie intake. However, this will only work if you don't overcompensate by eating larger meals when breaking your fast.

If you want to speed up the fat-burning and weight-loss process, then it is recommended that you eat a healthy low-carb diet in conjunction with fasting. This way, your body will remain in a fat-burning state for longer. Loading your body with carbs during your eating window will take your body a few steps backwards after you have endured a day fast.

Why should I intermittent fast if I don't need to lose weight?

Many choose to go the intermittent-fasting route as a lifestyle choice because of its added benefits. There are plenty of people who are reasonably slim and fit, yet they still choose to fast because they want to experience the healthy lifestyle choice that is associated with intermittent fasting. Here are some of the reasons why you should fast, regardless of you wanting to lose weight or not.

- Not only does it just improve brain function and mental sharpness but it also helps to prevent neurodegenerative diseases such as Alzheimer's and Parkinson's disease.

- It can naturally lower "bad" LDL cholesterol.

- It enables you to control your blood sugar levels better and can thus reduce the risk of you developing diabetes. It also helps diabetic patients by naturally decreasing insulin resistance.

- It can improve your body's ability to metabolize toxins.

- It reduces the body's oxidative stress levels. Oxidative stress is widely thought to increase the risk of heart disease and cancer, as well as diabetes.

- It can also reduce inflammation in the body, which is a key element in the development of many diseases.

- It has great potential to reduce the risk of chronic diseases and thus the potential to increase your overall lifespan.

- It automatically reduces your food and calorie intake, meaning less meals to prepare. If you begin preparing less food on a daily basis, you will begin to benefit from all that time saved from having to cook the meals that you will be skipping. You will also manage to save money this way. Every meal that you skip on a daily basis will add up as a monetary saving. Just imagine the cash you can potentially save over weeks and months.

- Studies have shown that fasting increases a person's brain function, which in turn increases their awareness and alertness. Fasting on a daily basis can certainly help you to be more energetic and sharper at work.

Chapter 5: Intermittent Fasting

Hacks and Tips

If you have taken part in regular intermittent fasts, then you may have hopefully noticed some form of weight loss as a result of the fast. This is actually quite a delicate phase of your new intermittent-fasting lifestyle because you can either get too excited by your weight loss and fall back into unhealthy eating, or you can get a good taste for your new weight-loss venture and look forward to taking things to the next level.

The results that you may have achieved thus far may seem great, but it is possible to still build upon those results without even spending that much more time in the gym or kitchen. You already have that intermittent-fasting mentality. Now it's time to improve upon that with some extra intermittent-fasting hacks and tips that will help you to take your new weight-loss regime to the next level.

Tip #1 Break Your Fast the Right Way

When you break your fast at the beginning of your eating window, you should stick to foods that will not cause your blood sugar to spike. The same goes for your insulin levels, which aren't something that remain consistent when you eat food. Intermittent fasting has been proven to assist in lowering insulin levels. Seeing that insulin is considered a fat-storage hormone, your body will, in fact, stop burning fat when your insulin levels become elevated.

It can become impossible to burn fat if there are large amounts of insulin present in your body. One of the main reasons for fasting is that it can help to burn fat because, as mentioned, fasting reduces insulin levels. However, if you complete a near-perfect fast that helped you achieve great insulin levels, only to eat the wrong food when breaking your fast, then you will cause your insulin levels and blood sugar to spike. When this happens, your body will actually begin to store fat instead of burning it.

If you want to keep the fat-burning process going, then it's best to stick to wholesome single- ingredient types of food when you break your fast. Most of these foods are positioned away from the other processed foods that you will find in a grocery store. Carbs are among the foods that have the most significant impact on your body's insulin levels. Some dairy products will also have a sizeable impact on your insulin, with protein having a moderate impact. Fat has the smallest effect on your insulin.

You can maintain decent insulin levels when breaking your fast if you do not overindulge in dairy or carbohydrates. A good hack for this is to consume as many vegetables as you can at breakfast so they will fill your stomach up while removing your hunger. After this, you can then move on to your protein and fat sources. If you still do feel hungry, then you can have some dairy or more fat. By doing this, you will be able to limit your insulin spikes during your eating window.

It's easy to get carried away and overdo it when you break your fast as you will have been thinking about eating food for a while. Try your best to limit yourself when you do eventually eat. If you find this difficult to do, then stick to the type of food as listed above.

Tip #2 Fast for Longer Periods

Because your fasting efforts will assist you in lowering your insulin levels, this will cause your body to burn fat for energy, meaning that that longer you fast, the more fat you can consume. When you feel you have mastered short-term intermittent-fasting protocols, you can then work your way up to extended fasting hours which can last you between 24 and 48 hours.

The 16/8 method requires you to fast for 16 hours a day. If you feel that 16 hours has become too easy for you and you are seeking out a real challenge, then ramp things up to 20 hours per day. There are people that swear by a 20-hour daily fast. They manage to accomplish this daily feat by shortening their eating window to just four hours. You can still spread out a couple of small meals in this short timeframe.

Once you have proven yourself with the four-hour eating window, you can then upgrade to OMAD status, which is One Meal A Day or what we mentioned as the Warrior Diet in an earlier section. This means that you will be fasting a full 24 hours, with just a single meal for the entire day. It doesn't end here. If you truly want to become an intermittent-fasting master, then you can push your fasting window up from 36 hours to 48 hours.

As with all of the fasting methods, the 36- to 48-hour fast may seem difficult and downright impossible to take on, but if you work your way to it and are ready for the challenge, then it can actually be easier than it looks. The more you get used to long periods of fasting, the more your fast will, in fact, blunt your hunger in such a way that it will actually feel like an appetite suppressant. Fasting for long periods of time like this will mean that your calorie consumption for the week will go down to a minimum. As mentioned earlier, long fasting hours mean longer fat- burning hours as well.

Tip #3 Fasting Workouts

Fasted workouts have not received much praise due to some findings from studies which claim that working out while you are fasting does not burn more calories than regular training during your eating window or within non-fasting individuals. One of the reasons for this is that most of these results have been flawed due to the fact most of the participants in those studies were given a meal-replacement shake right after their workout, which would have boosted their insulin levels.

There aren't that many studies focused on participants that continue to fast after training. Whatever the case may be, working out during or after your fast will help accelerate your fat burning as long as you keep to a good low-carb diet. Exercise can increase your appetite. Try your best to keep that appetite in check as you fast and train in the gym.

Tip #4 Strength Training

One of the fastest ways to completely deplete your glycogen stores in your body is to challenge your body by lifting heavy weights. Intense workouts with heavy weights will help bring your muscles close to failure. This sounds terrible, but your cells can rebuild to be much stronger afterward. This sort of training, combined with fasting, can assist in using up your current glycogen stores, as fasting is another excellent way of using up these glycogen stores.

By using up your glycogen fat stores, your body will then switch over to fat stores, which will trigger a fat-burning reaction. It's possible that weight training can also help you build more muscle, which will allow you to store more glycogen in your muscle cells instead of fat cells. If you are someone who is physically active, but you don't lift weights, it is advised that you do so. Try to start off small and slowly progress to heavier weights over time.

Tip #5 Avoid Artificial Drinks

Stay clear from energy drinks, soda, diet soda, juices, and other flavored beverages, even the ones that claim to be low in sugar as these drinks still contain plenty of artificial sweeteners that are not good for your health. Some of the negative ingredients in these drinks include Splenda, which can stimulate your appetite. It's best not to have any drinks with sugar, such as fruit juice, especially when you are fasting.

The best and safest plan is to drink plenty of water to keep yourself well hydrated. The great news about intermittent fasting is that it allows you to drink water as you fast, unlike other traditional and religious fasts. Intermittent fasting also allows you to have black coffee and tea, as well as herbal tea as long as there is no sugar or milk. Swap sugary sodas and juices for these alternatives that you can enjoy during and after fasting periods.

Tip #6 Keep Busy During Fasting Hours

This is a tip that is so close to the truth, to be genuinely successful when fasting: you should keep yourself busy during fasting windows. Keeping yourself busy with work or your favorite pastime or activity may keep your mind off food.

Anything, for that matter, that can distract you from thinking of food is best. In doing so, you will allow yourself the opportunity to adapt to fasting as well as help yourself develop that intermittent-fasting mentality that can help drive you to fast for more extended periods.

If you choose to start your fast in the evening, then you will spend most of your fasting window, if not a significant portion of it, asleep. This is why plenty of people begin their fasting window in the evening. Having your first meal between 10 a.m. and 12 p.m. may seem like a long stretch, especially if you are idle and have nothing better to do. Try and fill up your morning with some productive work to keep yourself busy before you break your fast. Those last few hours can become a handful while you patiently await your meal.

Tip #7 Sleep and Stress

Sleep is essential whether you take on intermittent fasting or not. It is crucial to our well-being and health as sleep assists us in repairing our bodies as well as helping us to lose weight. Your body will burn plenty of calories while you sleep, which will, in turn, assist in boosting your metabolism. Your body will undergo plenty of changes due to the fat burning that it will undergo from fasting. Rest up to ensure your body remains in good health.

One of the biggest triggers for overeating is stress. Many people stress-eat on a regular basis. And the food that people go for during stressful times is either unhealthy or full of carbs. The carbohydrates themselves won't help relieve the stress, but they help us endure stress because consuming carbs allows the brain to produce new serotonin. Serotonin actually makes us feel calmer; as a result, it makes us believe that we can cope. Avoid the trap and develop a healthy mindset that will allow you to control your stress while you are fasting and feasting.

Tip #8 Intermittent Fasting on a Ketogenic Diet

Most people who take on intermittent fasting usually practice balanced and flexible diets which have room for plenty of kinds of food. However, most diets focus on protein and have considerable amounts of carbs in them. Fasting will help you burn fat, while carbs will slow down this process. This means that you will be in and out of a fat-burning state. The keto diet promotes the fat-burning state of ketosis. Taking on the keto diet while fasting can help ensure that you remain in a constant fat-burning state.

If you want to begin the keto diet, then you will have to make sure that you consume the recommended macronutrients (minimal carbs with maximum fat). This can be seen as an effective way of feeding your body more fat for energy as your body is currently burning out all the fat. The "keto fast" has become a well-known dietary combination practiced by many people who are seeking outstanding results.

Tip #9 Don't Tell Anyone Who is Not Supportive

It's natural to seek out approval and support from your fellow peers. It is probably just as natural for your fellow peers to reject your ideas and your actions. It happens all too often: you start out a new venture in life and can't wait to tell everyone. Then the first person you speak to shoots down your new venture. This unneeded criticism is most likely not true, but you begin to feel discouraged.

Making changes in life is difficult. Starting out a new eating plan, like intermittent fasting, is a whole new lifestyle change that will leave you feeling awesome once you are fully into it. However, the hardest part, as with most things, is getting started. Gathering the willpower needed to start something new isn't easy as there is still so much doubt in your head. Now imagine a stranger, or even worse, a close friend shoots down your idea. It can leave you feeling depressed, which can cause you to abandon your new intermittent-fasting plan.

The thing is, those who do practice intermittent fasting love to share about it. So it can be difficult to contain yourself at times. But it is best to continue your fast on your own, without too many people knowing. At first. You should obviously tell your partner that you are taking part in intermittent fasting. Don't force your partner to join, though. This is your journey to fulfill.

Practice fasting during periods when you don't really have to socialize with people, like late at night and early in the morning. Reserve your eating window for times when you and your friends and family will most likely eat together. An example would be lunch and supper. This way, you won't have to explain intermittent fasting to people at a dinner table. You will risk the entire group going into a debate as to why should you or should not be fasting in the first place.

Try to find a good rhythm with your fasting and try and achieve excellent results first, before you begin to tell people. This way you will feel more comfortable when speaking to people who may wish to shoot down the idea or just debate with you. Who knows, the results that you achieve may be so great that people might start approaching you to ask you what your secret is.

Using Hand-to-Portion Food

Calorie counting has become the standard method of measuring our food consumption while offsetting it with the calories that we burn in a day. People say that the best way to lose weight is to count calories. To most, it's as simple as calories in vs. calories out. If you restrict your calorie intake to less than what you burn, then you will eventually lose weight. If you consume more calories than you can burn, then you will gain weight. However, when it comes to weight loss, it isn't that simple, and the same goes for counting calories.

When it comes to counting calories, you need to figure out how many calories are in the food you eat. This means you have to conduct plenty of research while taking down notes and figures related to the calories that you are eating. You will then have to add your figures up to make up your daily intake. There are quicker methods available, such as food-tracking apps like MyFitnessPal and Lifesum. However, even these apps don't know the exact calories in your food for sure.

The reason that these apps could give out wrong figures is that it is possible that the app and the research behind the figures are miscalculated, or you could have made an error while inputting the figures into the app. Research has shown that calorie databases can be out by 25 percent because of incorrect labeling, food quality, and other lab-related errors. There can even be significant variances among the different brands of foods. It's also easy to forget to write down some small snacks or sweets that you may have consumed on the fly.

There has been some praise recently given to new calorie and food measurement systems that depart from the normal calorie counting. One, in particular, does not consist of using measuring cups or scales, nor does it require smartphone apps or calculators. All you need is your hands. How it works is your palm determines for protein portions; your fist determines your vegetable portions; your cupped hand determines your carb portions; and your thumb determines your fat portions.

To determine your protein intake, you will need to use a palm-sized serving. This can be protein- dense food such as meat, fish, eggs, beans, or dairy. It is recommended that men have two palm-sized portions for each meal. One palm-sized portion of meat is recommended for women for each meal. It's important to remember that a palm-sized portion is the same thickness and diameter as your palm.

When it comes to your vegetable intake, it is recommended that men consume two fist-sized portions of vegetables with each meal. This applies to veggies such as spinach, broccoli, or carrots. For women, one fist-sized portion of veggies is recommended. The portion of vegetables must equal the same thickness and diameter as your fist.

You will use your cupped hands to determine the number of carbs you wish to consume. This is meant for carbohydrate-dense food such as starches, grains, fruits, etc. Two cupped hands are recommended for men while one cupped hand is recommended for women for most meals. With fat intake, its thumb-sized portions of fat-dense food such as butter, oil, nuts, and seeds. Two thumb-sized portions are perfect for men while one thumb-sized portion is right for women.

In general, the bigger you are, the bigger your hand is, the more you will need to consume. So not everyone will consume similar amounts as food. Your hand is your own personal measuring device for the food you wish to consume. Some people may confess to having large hands that are not proportionate to their body size. However, our hand size does somewhat correlate pretty closely with our general body size. This includes our muscle and bones.

Time- and Money-Saving Meal Prep

Making your meals from scratch at home takes up plenty of time and may not be as economical as you initially thought it would be. For this reason, most people would rather just eat out as it is convenient and, in some cases, cheaper. The problem with this is that you can quickly get caught up purchasing the wrong type of food, like high carb, unhealthy junk food. You also run the risk of upsizing your portions and overeating. Try reassessing your home cooking to prepare meals on the cheap quick and easy. Here are some tips below.

Tip #1 Keep Cooked Meat on Hand

Try cooking a whole bunch of meat or chicken in one go and then freezing it for later use. An example would be to prepare all of the chicken you just purchased from the grocery store as soon as you get home. You can then place your cooked chicken into small meal-sized portions (hand-measured, as explained above) into separate bags or freezer boxes. This way, you can merely defrost your meat the next time you wish to eat.

When you are eventually ready to eat, you can just remove a single meal-sized portion of the meat from your freezer, defrost, then heat up. You can cook your sides as you wait for your meat to defrost. This way you do not eat excessively, as you have already determined your portions. You will then only eat the portion that you defrost because you are obviously restricted here due to your earlier portion allocation. This way you will not over eat, or even waste food like before when you were not freezing your cooked meat. You would not waste as well if you did. It is a win-win situation.

Tip #2 One-Pot Meals

There will be times when you are not prepared to take on one of those quick-reheat dishes as you may have just run out of pre-cooked meat. An excellent quick and cheap solution for this scenario is to create a one-pot meals. Get together a whole lot of ingredients, throw them into a pot, and cook. There are plenty of great one-pot recipes out there that can even be made using a crock-pot. Having the ability to just throw everything together into a single dish, and you're done, means that meal prep will be kept as easy as possible and, in most cases, cheap.

Tip #3 Stock Up on the Essentials

It is absolutely crucial that you keep stock of your essential ingredients and food items at all times. If you find yourself missing a few simple ingredients, you may feel discouraged towards preparing your home-cooked meal. This might just be the thing to force you to go and eat take out again. The more you rely on cooking at home, the more you will be able to figure out the exact ingredients you need at all times.

You will even be able to pick up on which ingredients are running low so that you can make a grocery run and stock up. If you want to take things further, you can shop when your essential items are on sale. You can pick up your mayo and mustard in bulk when the prices are at rock bottom. This way you can ensure that you are fully stocked up on your essential items while saving on costs in the long run.

Tip #4 Cook in Double Batches

A great way to stretch your food a bit further is to cook in double batches. This means that instead of cooking just a single meal for yourself, you cook a larger portion that is twice as much. This way you can eat one portion that very evening and have the second portion later in the week. This works great if you cook yourself a lasagna. Baking a lasagna in the oven is no quick and easy feat. You can, however, bake once and eat twice.

This way you will get the most out of one cooking session. You can also freeze the remaining portions for use at a much later stage. This way you can even increase the portion size further and cook more than double. The excess food that you will not be able to be eating that evening can just go straight into the freezer.

Nutrient-Dense Food Swaps

There are many different types of food swap and substitution scenarios that can help you boost health while preventing disease. An example is bacon, which can itself be a meal. Bacon can also be a condiment, side dish, and even a dessert. Here are a few examples of fascinating swaps that you can implement into your daily diet and meal-prep routines.

Cauliflower Rice

Riced vegetables are becoming more popular. Not only do these vegetable-based rices allow us to easily consume the right amount of veggies, but they also serve as a great way to reduce our carb intake. Selecting rice cauliflower instead of rice in your food bowls can save you around 200 calories and carbs. It will also, in turn, increase the nutrient density of your meal.

Bean Chips

Bean-based chips are a new game changer in the munchies department that replaces the old- time favorite potato chips and pretzels. Bean-based chips also give you a significant boost in whole-food ingredients such as whole beans. Black bean chips have five grams of protein with only 85 mg of sodium and only ten digestible carbs. Try to stick to baked versions which go well with guacamole or even hummus.

Bean-Based Pasta

Bean-based pasta options are now becoming more available in the pasta aisles all around the world. In the past, the primary option was the healthy 100 percent whole-wheat version of pasta. Now, the nutritional figures totally favor the bean option.

Not only are they gluten-free, but bean-based pastas also contain about 20 grams more protein and eight grams more fiber. Bean pasta is also bound to fill you up faster than other traditional whole-wheat options. It is also a superb source of plant-based protein.

Ground Turkey or Tofu

Swapping ground beef for ground poultry means less saturated fat. This is good news for those who wish to keep their waistline intact. A recent study conducted in 2017 showed that too many unsaturated fats in a diet can possibly cause fat gain to your gut. Chicken breast and turkey meat are among the choices with the least amount of saturated fat.

Roasted Chickpeas

Eating plenty of salads can be seen as an excellent way to consume some low-calorie nutrients. However, even the best of salads can be flawed because of the inclusion of refined grains such as croutons. Swap out your croutons for delicious roasted chickpeas instead. You can either make them yourself or buy them. Including chickpeas in your salad can add fiber to your meal which can, in turn, assist in increasing your satiety while delivering healthy fats that can help metabolize your fat-soluble vitamins.

Sweet Potato Toast

Sweet potatoes are filled with antioxidants such as vitamin A and C, fiber, and potassium. Having this vegetable instead of bread can help you to reduce the grains in your diet while helping you to lose weight. Try it out for yourself by cutting a raw sweet potato into thin slices. You can do this by keeping the fiber-rich skin on. Toast until brown and then top as you would normally top a piece of toast. Some examples of toppings are avocado, eggs, cheese, etc.

Specific 5:2 Minimal Calorie Day Food Choices

With the 5:2 method of intermittent fasting, you will be required to fast for two nonconsecutive days in a week, while eating normally for the five remaining days. Most people try not to eat anything these days. However, you are allowed to consume around 500 calories each day. Five-hundred calories does not seem like much, and is perhaps less than a single meal for some people, but if planned correctly, you can manage a few small meals into the allotted 500 calories.

An example would be to have a small breakfast under 100 calories, lunch that is under 200 calories, and dinner which is between 200 to 300 calories. An example of a breakfast below 100 calories includes eating raisins, Greek yogurt, and almonds, which totals around 94 calories. Or you can opt for a spinach omelet that comes in at 94 calories as well.

Crushed new potatoes and shoots is a great lunch option that totals 170 calories. Or you could opt for a chicken miso soup which is a mere 12 calories. For dinner, you can have a simple vegetable chow mein (170 calories) or a Moroccan root tagine with couscous (238 calories). Small fruit snacks such as tangerines are great for in-between snacks to keep you going.

Conclusion

Thank you for absorbing the information found here. Hopefully, you were able to find all of the relevant information that you were looking for right here in these pages. This book has covered as much information as possible in regards to intermittent fasting. Information provided included the benefits of intermittent fasting and the science behind intermittent fasting.

The topic of intermittent fasting is very in depth as it covers various methods and ways in which you can begin your fasting journey as well as methods that are best suited for the more advanced. If you haven't started fasting yet, then try and make today your first day. Go ahead and abstain from food now, even if it is for just half a day. Do it regularly, and you will for sure reap the benefits.

Once your mindset has shifted to a more poised and balanced fasting mindset, then you will be able to handle long hours without food like a champ. If you are someone who doesn't care much for eating healthy, you can still fast. Because you have now become aware of your eating habits, you will automatically become aware of your eating. Hence, you might even adjust your food selection so that you can eat healthier.

The first few months might be a little difficult for you if you have never fasted before. Try easing into your fasts, as the book has suggested. Once you have progressed to someone who can fast for most of the day, try your utmost best to keep up with intermittent fasting. You will notice some real changes to your body and to your energy levels if you consistently fast for six months or more. Start fasting now and stick to it if you want to get the most out of intermittent fasting.

Good luck, and all the best on your intermittent-fasting journey.

P.S

If you have found any one thing of value or something which you have benefited from in this book, could I please seek your help once again to leave a review over in Amazon

It would be super helpful to let more folk know about what was the one thing that you learnt or benefited from

Thank You Very Much !

Made in the USA
San Bernardino, CA
31 January 2019